13/7/22

LIVING WITH HEARING LOSS AND DEAFNESS

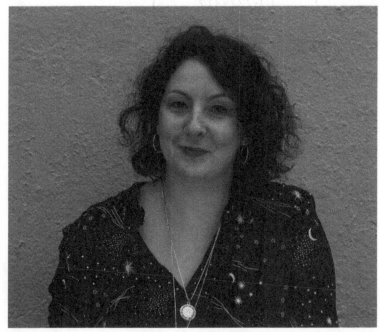

Samantha Baines is an award-winning comedian, actress, broadcaster and author. She is deaf, wears a hearing aid and is proud to be an Ambassador for the Royal National Institute for Deaf People. Her deaf activism includes TV and radio appearances, advising on campaigns, speaking to MPs at the House of Commons, raising money for deaf charities and fronting the RNID cinema subtitles campaign. Samantha has written two critically acclaimed children's books with deaf protagonists – *Harriet Versus the Galaxy* and *The Night the Moon Went Out*. She is a regular contributor on BBC radio and has written for publications including the *Guardian*, *Time Out*, *Huffington Post*, *Stylist Magazine* and the *Telegraph*. As an actress she has appeared in *The Crown*, *Call the Midwife* and *Silent Witness*, as well as hosting Magic Mike Live London in the West End.

www.samanthabaines.com

LIVING WITH HEARING LOSS AND DEAFNESS

Samantha Baines

First published in 2023 by Headline Home
an imprint of Headline Publishing Group

1

Cataloguing in Publication Data is available from the British Library

Trade paperback ISBN 978 1 0354 0150 5
eISBN 978 1 0354 0148 2

Publishing Director: Lindsey Evans
Senior Editor: Kate Miles
Copy Editor: Jane Hammett
Proofreaders: Nikki Sinclair and Anna Herve
Indexer: Ruth Ellis

Designed and Typeset by Avon DataSet Ltd, Alcester, Warwickshire

Printed and bound in Great Britain by Clays Ltd, Elcograf S.p.A.

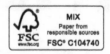

Headline's policy is to use papers that are natural, renewable and recyclable
products and made from wood grown in sustainable forests. The logging and
manufacturing processes are expected to conform to the environmental
regulations of the country of origin.

HEADLINE PUBLISHING GROUP
An Hachette UK Company
Carmelite House
50 Victoria Embankment
London EC4Y 0DZ

www.headline.co.uk
www.hachette.co.uk

Mum, thank you for buying me books for my birthdays.
I didn't always appreciate it then but I do now.
Thank you for believing in me.

Contents

Part 4: Support

Introduction

12 million people in the UK are currently living with hearing loss and deafness.

That's according to the Royal National Institute for Deaf People (RNID), and I'm their ambassador so I always get the most up-to-date stats. One of the perks of the job. You could also say it's 11,999,999 plus me, but I guess 12 million feels more succinct. RNID is all about connecting us – in fact, chief exec Mark Atkinson says: 'RNID is the only national charity that links together people who have all levels of hearing loss, the deaf community and people with tinnitus.' There you go.

We will explore many people's experiences of being deaf and hard of hearing in this book. My experience started as 'hearing loss', but many people I interview here were born deaf, communicate using British Sign Language (BSL), and have taught me what being deaf really means. Unless otherwise stated, all the quotes in this book come from interviews I have conducted. Thank you to everyone who gave me their time and agreed to be interviewed.

I became RNID celebrity ambassador (a volunteer role but, I mean, who do I think I am, calling myself a celebrity?) nearly

1

five years ago, and I have wanted to write this book for longer. I have two types of tinnitus; I have hearing loss in both ears; I wear a hearing aid on my right ear; I rely on lip-reading; I am learning BSL; and I call myself deaf. This is the book I searched for and couldn't find when I was told I needed a hearing aid. Mark says: 'Writing this book is important, because we know that hearing loss is something that is simply not talked about enough' – and he's a CEO and a white man so some people might be more inclined to listen to him. This book is not sponsored by RNID; I just like the organisation, and you'll soon find out why. As a self-deprecating (but working on it) comedian/actor/broadcaster/author and deaf queer woman, I thought I should give you some reasons to listen to me right up top.

Back to those stats, though: 12 million people with hearing loss and deafness? That's about 1 in 5 people in the UK. Look around you right now. Are you at work? On public transport? In a park? (If you are alone on the loo this bit won't work, so just picture it.) Find a group of around five people. Chances are, one of them has hearing loss, because that's how fractions work – and also I literally just told you that. One in five . . . so if we go by percentages, one of the Spice Girls could even become deaf. If it was Victoria, do you think she'd make designer hearing aids and send me some?

Chances are, one person in your family has hearing loss or is deaf. It might even be you. Two people in my family are deaf, because we're high-achievers. Yep, I have one hearing aid and my mum has two – she always has to go one better. You know mums! Seriously, though, it is lovely having a family member who knows what I'm going through, but when I was diagnosed with hearing loss (yes, that's the terminology medical professionals use) aged twenty-nine, it was a bit of a shock. Not even my mother could really help me with my feelings of premature ageing and 'otherness'. Turns out hearing loss isn't just for people with grey hair and Werther's Originals in their pockets – although, if that is you, I love you . . . and also please save me a sweet.

On my deaf journey I have met wonderful, interesting, cour-ageous people of all ages who also happen to be deaf, and I'm pleased to introduce you to a few of them in this book. Being involved with the deaf community is honestly one of the best bits about losing some hearing, and there is so much support out there if you know where to look. Luckily, working with RNID as their ambassador has introduced me to many people in this community, and I hope I can do the same for you here. This is an all-you-need-to-know book about hearing loss and deafness, with facts, experiences and words of wisdom from professionals. It's the book I wish I could have bought when the audiologist told me I needed a hearing aid, and I hope it can help you understand this new world you are stepping into. It's not a silent world; it's a busy, fascinating one.

'Basic deaf awareness goes a long way – make sure you face someone when you're talking, and repeat or rephrase informa-tion if the person doesn't understand you the first time. Don't make assumptions – instead ask what you can do to help,' advises Mark Atkinson. He is right, of course, and if you stop reading this book after the introduction then at least you will have absorbed that much. For me, basic deaf awareness isn't enough, and I think Mark would agree that we want to open the conversation around deafness: open it, dive into it and perform butterfly strokes across its sunlit waters. No more snorkelling; we are going to be deep-sea diving into hearing loss and deafness (and yes, I have been known to take a metaphor too far).

You might be reading this for yourself or on behalf of a loved one. Either way, thanks for taking an interest. I am a comedian, so it won't be a purely dry academic account of hearing loss and deafness; it will be . . . a flowery wet one? I'm honestly not sure what the opposite of dry academia is. I *will* share my experiences, good and bad, in the hope that they might help you, and I will speak to some other brilliant people about their experiences too. Let's laugh and learn together, shall we? Plus let's keep supporting each other, like a really excellent bra.

On average it takes TEN YEARS from noticing the first signs of hearing loss to actually doing anything about it. If that's you, well done for even getting here, for even picking up this book and reading the introduction. Ten years is the time it takes to see at least two UK prime ministers pass through government (more at the rate we are going), that's 5 billion 840 million miles the Earth will travel orbiting the sun, and that's about a fifth of the time it will take me to pay off my student loan. Wouldn't it be great if this book encouraged someone to get a hearing test? Or, after reading it, someone noticed that a family member might benefit from a lip-reading class? Or maybe it will help you – the person who has just been told they have hearing loss and are considering what that means for their future. Of course, if you were born deaf and are embedded in Deaf culture, you will already know much of this, but thank you for joining us on our journey.

When I was told I needed a hearing aid, I cried in a bike storage room at Westfield Shopping Centre. It was the only quiet place I could find at the time and I didn't really want to break down in the middle of H&M again (in my defence, their sizing is really weird). (I should say here that my audiologist is near Westfield; I didn't travel there purely to have a breakdown, like I was on a crying tour of the shopping centres of Britain.) I was completely shocked at my own hearing loss diagnosis. I was utterly unprepared to be a thirty-year-old deaf comedian, actor, writer and broadcaster. I worried that I would lose my job (whoever has heard of a deaf radio presenter?), that my life would become completely different, and that I would need a walking stick. I'm not sure why I suddenly imagined myself with a walking stick; we know that they don't aid hearing, but perhaps it was the idea that I was getting old before my time and that my body had already begun 'failing' me. All of this came crashing down on me in that bike storage room in Westfield, and so I rang my mother and cry-mumbled to her until a bewildered cyclist walked in on my teary saga.

You may not have had as climactic a 'diagnosis moment' as I did, but it may have still been a difficult one. You may have been born deaf and grown up coming to terms with an ableist society forcing you to live in a hearing world. You may even have breezed through all of it and only felt its impact later, like a hot curry. Whatever your journey, the first – and most important – thing you need to know is that you are not on your own. There are 11,999,999 people in the UK – plus me – who can relate to what you're going through. Unfortunately I couldn't get in contact with all of them for this book, as I had a deadline, but knowing they are out there is nice. No matter how 'strange' or 'other' or 'broken' you might feel right now (and, trust me, I felt all of those things), we're all in this together and I'm here to remind you that you are not 'broken'; you are wonderful and loved and you are deaf. Yes, even if the audiologist tells you that you have 'hearing loss', you are allowed to call yourself 'deaf'. Deafness can actually be a strength: it can change your life for the better like it has mine (plus you will get a third off public transport, cheap tickets at the theatre, and can listen to Britney songs via your hearing aid without anyone knowing).

Welcome to the deaf club.

You said you're a comedian – is this a joke to you?

Me: 'I have hearing loss . . .'

Stranger: 'What? Ha ha, get it!?'

That is a deaf joke, but please DO NOT – I repeat, DO NOT – EVER MAKE THIS JOKE. If you have been on the receiving end of people making this joke *at you* over and over again, you have my deepest sympathies. We (the hearing loss/deaf community) hear it all the time, and it's not very creative or very clever.

When you dig a bit deeper into it, the 'what?' joke is basically a stranger saying 'I don't know what to say, so I'm going to make a joke to show that I'm fine with it'. I always feel like saying in response, 'I'm sorry you feel awkward, but leave the jokes to me, babe.' I always add 'babe' because it sounds particularly condescending and patronising, which can be useful in this situation. I think it was Jane Austen who wrote, 'It is a truth universally acknowledged . . . that you shouldn't make a joke about something unless you have experienced that thing.' Well, she probably thought it, even if she didn't say it. Deaf people can make the 'what?' joke because then it's an informed joke. We have hearing loss/deafness, we have experienced its ups and downs, and that comes with some joke permissions.

Usually if someone is disclosing their deafness to you, it is for a reason. Perhaps they want to let you know why they can't hear you, they want to explain their hearing aid, indicate how best to communicate with them, or they want to let you into their lives. And none of those scenarios warrants a joke as a response.

'Er . . . Sam, aren't you a comedian? Don't you love a joke?!' Yes, fair point, but discovering you are deaf isn't funny at the time. It can be shocking, isolating and confusing. However, during some of the most challenging times in our lives it is humour that gets us through, because life can be ridiculous and hilarious. Deafness can be challenging; not *being* deaf, but the way society makes deafness a challenge, through stigma, ageism and inaccessibility.

Humour helps me work through new information, my ever changing identity, and difficult experiences. Being deaf isn't funny, but some of the encounters it leads to, memories it stirs, and experiences I have had are funny, and I've included some of those in this book. There are also some incredible facts, well-researched quotes and even several opinions.

Part 1
All about deafness

Chapter 1

Terminology around deafness: am I deaf?

You might be reading this book and thinking, 'Am I deaf?' Well, the answer to this question can be both straightforward and complicated. Sounds fun, eh? The simplest answer is yes. If you do not have full hearing, as determined by a professional audiologist using a hearing test, then yes, you are part of the deaf community. However, there is much debate among the deaf community about what deaf individuals should call themselves. Also, hearing people don't always know how to describe their deaf counterparts.

I have used 'hearing loss' in this book, as that is usually how it's described in a medical environment. Because of this, 'hearing loss' is the term that people new to this journey will relate the most to. I don't love the 'loss' connotations (explained on p. 16), which is why I use the terms 'deaf' and 'deafness'. These are more accepted within the deaf community.

In short, people have many different views on the terminology to use around deafness, and will tell you about their views at length, when prompted (and sometimes without being prompted) on social media. So what terminology should you use? I'm going to answer this question using my experience and from the information I have received from interviewing experts and people with different deaf experiences.

'Am I disabled?' is another question that comes up around this topic, and we will delve into that on p. 255.

Deaf categories

First, the science. There are widely recognised categories of hearing loss and deafness, and these are based on the results of your hearing test. The British Society of Audiology lists these categories on its website:

- **Normal hearing:** You can hear quiet sounds of less than 20 dBHL (although it is possible to have hearing difficulties even if your hearing is in this range).
- **Mild hearing loss:** Hearing loss between 20–40 dBHL (typically you might find that you have difficulty following speech in noisy situations).
- **Moderate hearing loss:** Hearing loss between 41–70 dBHL (you will probably find that you have difficulty following speech).
- **Severe hearing loss:** Hearing loss between 71–95 dBHL (you will have severe difficulty following speech without a hearing aid).
- **Profound hearing loss:** Hearing loss over 95 dBHL (you may have need of hearing aids, cochlear implants, sign language and lip-reading).[1]

dB = decibels HL = hearing loss

Let's ignore the word 'normal'. I've never liked to be 'normal' anyway. I would rather call that category 'full hearing'. I have moderate hearing loss, which I would call medium in layman's terms. If Starbucks made hearing loss, I'd be a tall latte with oat milk. 'Short' would be mild hearing loss, 'tall' is moderate, 'grande' is severe and 'venti' is profound, in case you find that easier to remember. (The oat milk is just because I am dairy-intolerant.) 'Stone deaf', a term that popped into existence in 1762, is no longer widely used – although you may not be surprised to hear that someone used the phrase in front of me very recently. It means 'completely deaf' or, as we would refer to it in the deaf community, 'profoundly deaf'. However, being profoundly deaf doesn't always mean an absence of sound, as Annie Harris, RNID advocacy officer and BSL user, explains: 'I wish people realised that deaf does not always mean silence.' In fact, even people who are profoundly deaf might not experience complete silence, so that's a myth that we need to bust straight away.

It is important to note that of the 12 million people with hearing loss and deafness in the UK, 10.3 million have mild to moderate hearing loss. That means over 85 per cent of the deaf population in the UK have small to medium hearing loss. Therefore the majority of people in the UK do not fall into the 'profoundly deaf' and 'users of sign language' categories, as many hearing people might assume. However, it is important to note that it's not just profoundly deaf people who know and use sign language; everyone is welcome!

So, are you deaf? Yes and no. Some people prefer to call themselves capital D Deaf. Usually this community express a pride in their status and don't see themselves as having 'lost' anything or as 'suffering' in any way. It is important to note that many people who call themselves lower-case deaf also feel this. The capital D deaf community is an historical one: it includes those who are born Deaf, those who are born into a Deaf family, and/or those whose main method of communication is British Sign Language. This community truly and factually haven't lost anything, as hearing has never been an important part of their lives. You see, you can't miss something you have never had. Of course, being Deaf goes further than this, as it has its own culture, traditions and language. Today there is a movement within the capital D Deaf community promoting the use of the lower-case d deaf descriptor to include more of the wider deaf community, but this is a personal choice. For consistency, I will use deaf with a lower-case d throughout this book.

Terminology can be scary. If you're talking to or being introduced to a deaf person, the best thing to do is ask how they see themselves and how they'd like you to refer to them. Deaf people are humans too, so we get it. There are some general guidelines below, but terminology in deafness, just like in sexuality ('Oh hi, I'm bisexual too') is a very personal thing, so there will always be exceptions to the rule. As Amy Morton, founder of organisation Living with Hearing Loss, puts it, 'There is no "one size fits all" with hearing loss' – and there is very rarely a 'one size fits all' in T-shirts either, despite what internet sites will try and tell you.

Hearing-impaired

You would be surprised by how many educational settings have a 'hearing-impaired unit', even though this is considered very old-fashioned language today. I guess change happens slowly in the education system. After all, BSL is still rarely offered as a language option in schools, and is not part of the curriculum. Deaf journalist and activist Liam O'Dell describes 'hearing-impaired' as 'an outdated term to describe a deaf person', and I would agree. Many people in the deaf community do not like to be called hearing-impaired, as it has very negative connotations. 'Impaired' is a loaded word: as a deaf person, I feel that it is not my hearing loss that impairs me but society's lack of accessibility.

Keighley Miles leads a local support group called Families of Deaf Children (FDC) in Essex. She explained how she feels about the term:

> Growing up, I always said I was hearing-impaired or hard of hearing, quickly followed by 'But I can hear and talk!' Now I can't stand the term 'hearing-impaired', and have actually got the council to launch a consultation to change the local schools in Essex that use the name within their resource base. This was a success, and the names are in the process of being changed.

See, one person can make a difference – thanks, Keighley! People who use the phrase 'hearing-impaired' to describe themselves should not be shunned, though; they will usually have been introduced to the phrase through a hearing lens (views held by someone who comes from a hearing environment and background, so their views are highly influenced by the fact that hearing for them is the 'norm' and they have no experience of a world in which not hearing is the 'norm'. This is a similar concept to white privilege) and who may not know its connotations. The best thing is to make sure that a person has all the terminology information they need through a deaf lens too (i.e. informed by the knowledge of a deaf person) so they can make an informed decision about how to describe themselves. Remember, for decades people didn't have access to all the information we have today at our fingertips on the internet, or access to the wider deaf community, and that's not their fault. They may still choose to call themselves hearing-impaired, and that's okay!

Hearing loss/hard of hearing

'Hearing loss' and 'hard of hearing' are terms generally used in the UK to describe people who are born with full or some hearing and then lose their hearing over time. These people, including me, are part of the wider 'deaf community' (generally written as deaf with a small d).

I use the term 'hearing loss' in this book, although I know that not all the deaf community identify with this, as they don't like the use of the word 'loss'. But 'hearing loss' seems more scientific to me than 'hard of hearing', and I've always loved science and had a bit of a crush on Brian Cox. As it's a fact that I have lost some hearing that I used to have, it seems correct to me – and, as a happily divorced woman, I know loss isn't always a bad thing! Saying that, nowadays I choose to call myself deaf. The term 'hard of hearing' doesn't resonate with me because of the word 'hard', which suggests it's something I need to work at, just like exams are hard. However, Amy Morton says: 'I identify as hard of hearing: however, depending on the conversation, I will say I have a severe hearing loss in both ears or I am severely deaf in both ears.' So you see, it really is a personal thing!

Rita Kairouz, audiologist and founder of Little Auricles, agrees:

Everyone is different. Some people prefer to be called deaf while others prefer hard of hearing and some even say they are hearing-impaired or disabled. I tend to use deaf and hard of hearing as I feel these terms are more positive and don't further stigmatise the community.

Hearing-aid wearer

Some prefer to categorise themselves based on physical additions, such as hearing aids. 'Hearing aids' usually covers devices from in-ear hearing aids, which sit completely inside the ear, much like the earpieces worn by TV presenters, to over-the-ear hearing aids which are a bit like a discreet Bluetooth headset that wraps around the back of the ear. There are also cochlear implants, which are attached to the side of the head under general anaesthetic, as well as other types of aids. It is important to note that not all hearing loss/deafness can be helped by a hearing aid or cochlear implant. If someone tells you they are deaf, suggesting that they try hearing aids is not always helpful, as they may have tried them previously and had had no luck with them. Another important point is that hearing aids do not 'cure' or 'fix' deafness. Deafness cannot be reversed, and many deaf people don't appreciate talk of a 'cure', as this implies that deafness is some sort of disease that *needs* to be 'cured', which of course it is not. So hearing aids cannot reverse your deafness: however, they can utilise and amplify the hearing you do have, which helps some people. We look at hearing aids in depth in Chapter 5.

I have an over-the-ear hearing aid, which I love. It helps me in noisy environments by dulling background noise, it amplifies sounds, and importantly, it also streams music and podcasts! If I ever look a bit vacant during a conversation, I'm usually listening to Beyoncé. I also use the phrase 'I am a hearing-aid wearer' as this is factual, clear, and lets others know that I have communication needs.

Lip-reader

Another physical categorisation is saying 'I am a lip-reader.' Many people like this terminology as it not only suggests deafness but it also indicates how the person will be listening (by reading your lips), which is useful for the speaker. Lip-reading teacher and lip-reader herself Lisa Cox says: 'Just say "I need to lip-read you." It is very successful. It is positive, as it says what I *can* do and makes it clear what I need – very useful when someone is wearing a mask.'

If someone lip-reads it is important to face them while you are talking, keep your mouth visible (e.g. don't cover it with your hand) and speak normally. Over-enunciation actually makes lip-reading harder, so please avoid that when speaking to lip-readers. You don't have to be Julie Andrews for us to understand you.

It can be harder to lip-read when you meet someone for the first time, as an accent may alter the way their mouth moves and different people use different speech patterns. We will look further into this in Chapter 8.

Deaf

As mentioned, Deaf (with a capital) is generally reserved for people with profound hearing loss, usually from birth. As Deaf actor Sophie Stone puts it: 'I was born Deaf so I don't consider myself to have "lost" anything . . . no loss, no impairment, not failed or broken.'

People who use BSL as their first language can also call themselves Deaf. RNID advocacy officer Annie Harris agrees: 'I am Deaf, because as well as my profound deafness, I consider myself to be part of the deaf community, where we communicate using BSL, which is a beautiful, rich language.' Sophie Stone agrees: 'I'm Deaf. Big D Deaf because I've found my identity, my truth and community.'

Some activists are pushing for the whole of the deaf community to be recognised under one term, using either 'Deaf' or 'deaf', but this is not yet widely accepted in the UK. As Clare-Louise English, co-founder of and co-artistic director at Hot Coals Productions, puts it:

> I liked using 'small d deaf', which used to be common, because for me it spoke to the fact that I consider myself as deaf and part of the community but without claiming I'm something I'm not, because I wasn't born deaf with BSL as my first language. Nowadays, though, people prefer to use 'big D Deaf' for everyone, which is more inclusive, though I think we've lost some of the nuance of d/Deaf.

Many within the BSL community want to preserve their beautiful language and Deaf culture, and recognising everyone who has some degree of deafness or hearing loss may cause this to be lost. American model and activist Nyle DiMarco says, 'the capital D is a choice. It is how I see myself, and how I want to be seen. It's my preferred way of naming my identity'.[2]

deaf

The 'deaf community' (lower-case d) generally covers a whole range of hearing experience. Personally, I love to use 'deaf', as it feels inclusive of those with mild/moderate hearing loss, those who lip-read and use subtitles, those with hearing aids/ cochlear implants, and those who use BSL – without blurring our experiences. So often we only see extreme impressions of deafness represented on mediums such as TV – for example, the baby on YouTube getting a hearing aid and hearing their mother's voice for the first time, or Grandad who won't turn his hearing aids on, so the whole family has to shout. It is important to note that these examples do not reflect the majority of the deaf community, who are thriving, even when society tries to make everyday life particularly inaccessible. Remember, 1 in 5 people in the UK have some form of deafness. That is 12 million people in the UK, 10.3 million of whom have mild to moderate hearing loss (stats from RNID, 2022). Yes, many of these people are over sixty, but that doesn't mean they are the grandad who won't turn his hearing aids on. Many people will never tell anyone about their deaf status, while others prefer not to use hearing aids or choose to ignore the signs of hearing loss. That is their decision.

Interior designer Micaela Sharp says: 'I always say I'm "partially deaf in one ear" so that people understand they need to speak up.' However, when it comes to how deafness affects her life, 'Most of the time I completely forget about it.'

I wrote this book to help inform readers, but not to shame anyone for their personal choices around their deaf experience. You do you! No matter where you are in your deaf journey, it is never too late to find a community, if you feel inclined to. Keighley Miles, leader of FDC, says: 'Make connections with the deaf community even if you don't identify as deaf. You will be surprised how many people don't feel they fit into the deaf category.'

I know I didn't feel comfortable calling myself 'deaf' at the beginning, but that changed over time, just like it did for

Keighley: 'Now I identify as deaf because when I take off my cochlear processor I hear nothing.'

Outside the UK

If you thought the above was complicated, well, there are nuances in terminology outside the UK too. Jenni Ahtiainen, founder of hearing-aid jeweller company Deafmetal, explains: 'In Finland, "deaf" and "hard of hearing" have a huge difference. The groups do not want to mix with each other. But in English outside Finland I generally consider myself to be part of the deaf community, although I am hard of hearing.' In America the use of Deaf is also more pronounced, and is promoted by many Deaf institutions.

So what have we learned?

British Sign Language teacher Fletch@ summarises it pretty well:

> Hearing loss means you are hearing but you start to lose your hearing. Deaf means you are profoundly Deaf and you are very proud to be Deaf within the Deaf world. [Lowercase] d-deafness means you are deaf but you are within the hearing world and adapt to the hearing world.

As we have discovered in this chapter, terminology around this is tricky, and no one phrase works for everyone. As RNID chief exec Mark Atkinson says:

> Everyone's experience of deafness or hearing loss is different, and it's important not to put people in a box. Everyone has a

different story – some people are born deaf, while others lose their hearing as a result of noise exposure or a genetic condition. Everyone has different communication needs – some people use BSL, others lip-read or use subtitles. As a hearing person, it's important to listen and learn how you can support someone and not make assumptions.

The best thing to do is be led by the individual and ask how they like to describe themselves. If you are just starting your deaf journey, I hope the above descriptions have helped, but at the end of the day you should use whichever term resonates most with you. It is *your* deaf experience and no one else can tell you how to live your life – well, except our mothers, and our therapists, and our best friends on a night out – but you get the idea.

In this book I will use the phrase 'deaf' to describe all experiences of deafness, but please insert your preferred terminology when reading.

Chapter 2
Why am I deaf?

Many people are born deaf. Some choose not to use hearing aids, and still live full, glorious lives. Other people are born with full hearing and then lose some of their hearing over time, like me. This chapter talks about the people like me and our experiences, as well as looking more closely at the reasons people become deaf. For clarification, I will refer to my deafness as hearing loss in this chapter. Lots of research is being done to try to discover the causes of hearing loss so it can be prevented: however, some people in the deaf community see this research as trying to eradicate the deaf community.

According to a World Health Organization (WHO) report from 2021, 'In children, nearly 60 per cent of hearing loss is due to avoidable causes that can be prevented through implementation of public health measures. Likewise, in adults, most common causes of hearing loss, such as exposure to loud sounds and ototoxic medicines, are preventable.' The report goes on to state that, across the world: 'By 2050 nearly 2.5 billion people are projected to have some degree of hearing loss and at least 700 million will require hearing rehabilitation.'[3]

Hearing loss is not something that is going away, and it's desperately important that we talk about it.

When I was born in the late 1980s (I know! I read younger, right?!), babies were not given hearing tests as standard. This makes me wonder: if I had a hearing test as a newborn, what would it have shown? As a child, I had many ear infections, and even then I don't remember my hearing being checked. If I had a hearing test at birth or in my early years, would it have detected some loss? If I had found out about my deafness at a younger age, I would have been able to learn so many more skills that would definitely help me today – BSL, for example. And if I knew I had hearing loss, perhaps I would have looked after my ears a little better at concerts as a teenager.

As soon as I discovered I had hearing loss, in my late twenties, my next question was: why? Why has this happened? Did I do something wrong? I also needed to know from an emotional standpoint: I had this new diagnosis, but finding out a reason for it would make it solid and real, help me accept it. If there wasn't a reason for it, I thought, then maybe it was all just a big mistake.

Audiologist and founder of hearing-aid jewellery company Little Auricles Rita Kairouz says: 'There is a wide range of reasons for a potential hearing loss, and some are curable. Your audiologist and ENT specialist will be able to work out exactly what is wrong and why.' Curable reasons include ear infections and ear wax build-up. However, if you are diagnosed with medical hearing loss, like I was, this is not reversible. Nothing will make your hearing better again, but there are things that will help you, such as BSL, the deaf community, and possibly hearing aids.

If you have a sudden loss of hearing, you should contact your GP immediately.

Hereditary deafness

Yes, much like dairy intolerance or a strong sense of self-worth, deafness can be passed down from your parents. Thanks, Mum. My mum has hearing loss, and uses two hearing aids, as well as being dairy intolerant and having a strong sense of self-worth – it's quite the inheritance for me! Luke Christian, owner of clothing brand Deaf Identity, has an even stronger inheritance: 'I was born deaf and it is genetic in my family, going back at least eight generations.'

The Royal National Institute for Deaf People's website explains that:

> A dominant gene mutation that causes hearing loss can come from the mother or the father. The chance of passing on this mutation to your children is one in two . . . A recessive gene mutation that causes deafness in a child must have been passed on by both the mother and father. If the child only inherits one copy of the affected gene from one parent, they'll be a carrier. This means that although they can hear, they can pass on the affected gene to their own children.[4]

A 1 in 2 chance of passing on the gene, eh? Yes, I do have one sister – and no, she doesn't have hearing loss. Maths in action!

In contrast, illustrator Lucy Rogers was:

> Born deaf to hearing parents, so at first my parents were not quite sure what was happening as I was their first baby, but they knew something wasn't right as I didn't look up whenever someone said my name . . . My parents were a bit worried, obviously, about raising a deaf child, but luckily I had a great

25

audiologist who assured them it would be okay and to communicate with me in SSE (so both sign language and spoken English) so I could pick up both.

Lucy's deafness could have been caused by recessive genes in both parents, or by another cause.

Noise-induced hearing loss

This is hearing loss caused by exposure to loud sounds. These sounds can be for a short period of time, like a gunshot close to your ear, or a long period of time, like working continuously in a loud environment like a factory or as a party planner for hen dos. Age-related hearing loss can also fall into this category, due to noise exposure over the years.

Sound is measured in decibels (dB), just like electrical current is measured in volts or health is measured in Instagram posts of smoothies and yoga poses. Decibels sound Christmassy, which I like. It makes me think of the bells of December that Santa's elves get out every year to mark the start of that tinsel-fuelled month. Anyway, it just means how loud something is.

Sounds over 85 dB, heard for a prolonged period, can be harmful to humans. How loud is that? Well, 85 decibels could be a very noisy restaurant with music, laughter and clanging of dishes. Yes, socialising could cause hearing loss! A great excuse for not going out to that work colleague's birthday, right?!

Did you know that legally you can't work in an environment where the sound level is over 85 decibels without hearing protection? Really, waiting staff and bar people should be wearing hearing protection, just like musicians do at concerts.

If you are unsure if an environment is too loud, RNID provide this useful example on their website: 'In a real-life situation, you should be able to talk to someone who is 2 metres away without having to shout over background noise. If you can't be heard over the background sounds, the noise level could be hazardous.' You can also download free apps for your phone that measure sound levels, if you want to work out exactly how many decibels you are being exposed to.

Hearing loss caused by noise usually results in an initial loss of the higher frequencies. This will then spread to other frequencies if the exposure continues. My hearing loss was originally in the higher frequencies, which means goodbye to birdsong, some doorbells and my watch alarm. Hence the reason I'm always late, miss all my packages, and forget birds exist. When I discovered that noise could be the cause of my hearing loss, I immediately blamed the band Limp Bizkit, even though there is absolutely no proof it has anything to do with them. I do, however, remember going to their concert aged thirteen or so and sitting near a huge speaker because those were the cheap seats. My friends seemed to be having an excellent time, but I had gone along despite hating the band because I wanted to like the same things that my friends did. I remember it being very loud and shouty. Fred Durst (the lead singer) was singing 'Keep rollin', rollin', rollin'', which was my favourite of all their songs, and I was counting down the minutes until I could get back out into the quiet night air and roll on home. Years later, I was not shocked to find out that Fred Durst himself has hearing loss, and it has been reported that he now uses American Sign Language to communicate. Sending you lots of love, Fred.

Eardrum damage

When I do talks for children and ask 'Why might someone lose their hearing?', I am surprised to discover that the first thing a child suggests is always a burst eardrum. Many people assume that hearing loss needs to be caused by an extreme event (like a noise being so loud it bursts your eardrum), but the gradual effect of noise has just as big an impact. Eardrum damage tends to come under noise-induced hearing loss; however, things like infections and even a bad ear wax removal process can also damage your eardrum. Avoid unregistered ear-wax removal practitioners!

Infections/diseases

Infections when you are in the womb can lead to hearing loss, as can birthing complications including 'birth asphyxia (a lack of oxygen at the time of birth), hyperbilirubinemia (severe jaundice in the neonatal period), low birth weight, other perinatal morbidities and their management'.[5] Meningitis, glue ear and chronic ear infections in childhood can also be a cause, as can viral infections and chronic diseases in adulthood. Some infections can lead to damage or a burst eardrum, or a medication to treat a certain condition may have the side effect of hearing loss (see the section on ototoxic drugs on p. 30). Author Jaipreet Virdi explains the cause of her deafness in her book *Hearing Happiness: Deafness Cures in History*: 'When I was four years old, I became ill with bacterial meningitis and nearly died',[6] whereas interior designer Micaela Sharp explains: 'I was about thirty-two and woke up one day to discover I couldn't hear fully out of one ear. I'd had a virus, so I thought my ear was blocked.' She discovered that she had significant hearing loss on one side. It could have been the virus that caused the loss, or perhaps it just exacerbated a loss that was already there. Sudden hearing loss is not very common, and it is important to book an appointment with your GP or audiologist straight away if this happens.

Two well-known diseases cause hearing loss and tinnitus: labyrinthitis and Ménière's disease. However, blogger Bethan Harvey explains there are other rarer conditions that don't fall under diseases that can cause deafness too:

> I was born with microtia, which is a rare condition affecting 1 baby in every 7,000. I was born with grade 3 microtia to my right ear, meaning I was born with a peanut-sized fold of skin tissue with no ear opening instead of the typical 'normal' ear with cartilage and opening. As a result, I was born fully deaf with no hearing in my right ear.

Ear wax

One of the few causes of hearing loss that is curable is ear wax. You may have a wax build-up, in which case you need to see an audiologist, who can remove it safely – and possibly restore your hearing. Wax is one of the first things a GP or audiologist should check before giving you a hearing test. Wax build-up is pretty common, but you can no longer get ear wax removal services on the NHS; you will have to pay for this in the UK.

As audiologist Adam Chell advises, 'The general rule is, don't put anything in your ear that is smaller than your finger.' Please don't try and get around that by using your child's finger – that is gross, but excellent creative thinking. Using cotton buds to remove wax can actually make your wax problems worse.

Adam has also removed the tips of cotton wool buds from patients' ears, so be warned! Using a few drops of olive oil in your ear overnight to dislodge wax is generally considered a safe home remedy. But if you suspect you may have a burst eardrum, do not use olive oil as it could cause further damage.

Menopause

Unfortunately, as with many health conditions that affect women, there hasn't been enough study into the relationship between menopause and hearing loss.[7] However, an American study in 2013 concluded that 'Older age at menopause [over 50] and longer duration of postmenopausal HT [hormone therapy] are associated with higher risk of hearing loss.' It would be great to see more studies into this connection, but it's worth being aware of if you are going through the menopause and notice symptoms of hearing loss.

Ototoxic drugs

Powerful drugs like those used to treat cancer can cause hearing loss. Some types of penicillin can also cause hearing loss, but only in large doses. Speak to your GP if you have any worries. Some antibiotics also cause hearing loss: 'The group of antibiotics that is most likely to cause hearing loss is called aminoglycosides. These include gentamycin, streptomycin, neomycin. These antibiotics are often used to treat serious or life-threatening bacterial infections such as tuberculosis'.[8]

There is little reported connection between recreational drugs and hearing loss, but some studies have claimed that opioid addiction (heroin, morphine, fentanyl) can cause hearing loss. I wonder if a study has been carried out yet on the connection between cannabis and hearing loss? If not, I'm sure that lots of people in cafés in Amsterdam would be interested in taking part.

Brain tumours

Yes, this is what came up on Google when I looked up causes for my hearing loss. I have anxiety, and I really should have learned by now not to google symptoms . . . I should just wait to see a doctor. However, because my hearing loss was one-sided and I had loss in the higher frequencies, I was sent for an MRI to check I didn't have a brain tumour. You can imagine how anxious I was waiting for that appointment. I was actually writing a stand-up comedy show at the time, and being told I might have a brain tumour was not conducive to being creative – or funny. I blamed every badly written joke on my possible brain tumour. The brain scan itself was fine, as long as you aren't claustrophobic, although it's – ironically – very loud and they play music over the top of the machine noise in an attempt to drown it out, so if you have any sort of noise sensitivity, which I do, then the whole thing is quite intense.

You have to remove all metal from your body before you have an MRI as it's basically a huge magnet, and you absolutely spend the first ten minutes worrying you haven't accidentally swallowed a nail. You also have to take off your bra, as they can have metal underwiring, which I remember being really prudish about. I guess I never expected to get to second base with a machine. When the ordeal is finally over, you are led back to your bra (and your clothes) and you gaze deeply into the eyes of the healthcare worker escorting you, wondering if they are treating you like you have a brain tumour. You know the people on the other side of the MRI screen have seen your scan and know whether it is clear or not, but you have to wait a couple of weeks for a doctor to tell you the result.

Here are some facts that I, due to extreme anxiety, paid a private doctor to tell me while I was waiting for my MRI scan and results. The most common type of tumour that can cause hearing loss is called an acoustic neuroma. These grow on the nerve used for hearing and balance, so can lead to hearing loss and being unsteady on your feet. Acoustic neuromas are benign (non-cancerous) and usually very small. If you have a small acoustic neuroma, healthcare staff will likely just monitor it and leave you to get on with your daily life. Only if the tumour is very large and causing extreme problems would they operate to remove it. Luckily, acoustic neuromas tend to grow very slowly, so many people don't need treatment.

The most important fact the expensive private doctor told me was that 'acoustic neuromas are estimated to affect about 1 in 100,000 people in the general population' (as quoted by the National Organisation for Rare Disorders).[9] That fact was worth every penny of his consultation fee, to be honest. He calmed my nerves, and eventually I was told that my MRI scan was clear.

No idea

Unfortunately this is a very common answer to the question 'what caused my hearing loss?' Often a possible reason can be identified as a cause of hearing loss or deafness, but it can be hard for medical professionals to be sure. In fact, I have no definite answer to that question myself. As I mentioned, my mum has hearing aids, so my deafness could be hereditary or due to a combination of ear infections and noise damage, but I will never know. I have never received a reason from an audiologist as it is so difficult to determine. Initially, this can be hard to accept and deal with. Being told you have hearing loss feels like such a huge life event, so not knowing why it has happened can feel unnerving. It can feel good to have something or someone to blame, whether this is your parents or an unsuspecting 1990s rock band, but the cause doesn't change your new reality.

Learning to accept – and even own – my new deaf status, and finding ways to make my everyday life easier, were important steps for me in coming to terms with my hearing diagnosis. I really value the fact that my friends in the deaf community accept their deafness as part of them and have pride in their community. This gave me a goal to work towards. Exploring the impact my hearing loss would have on my life, as I do in this book, helped me see that practical solutions and help were available.

Chapter 3
The first signs

The beginning of your deaf journey can be very different depending on your experience and upbringing. Deaf actor Sophie Stone says: 'As I was born deaf, I don't know myself any other way. I didn't have worries or feel different from anyone else until I saw how other parents and people spoke to each other. I was also bullied and hearing aids seemed alien to people.' Sophie's first sign that she was different to her peers was how other people reacted to her. British Sign Language teacher and performer Fletch@ has a similar memory:

> When I was eleven, I had a form to complete in secondary school. One question asked if I was deaf or hearing. I ticked the box for hearing. The teacher said, 'No, you're not hearing, you're deaf.' I said, 'No, I'm hearing, I can hear music, all sounds etc.'. She said, 'No, you're deaf, you're wearing hearing aids.' That's when I found out, and I was confused, but not worried, at that time.'

As Fletch@ describes, terminology can be confusing for young people, especially if no one explains deafness to them or if they come from a hearing family with no experience of deafness. Fletch@ could hear some sound with her hearing aids, so she assumed she wasn't deaf, as her perception of deafness was an absence of all sound. However, from the perspective of a hearing teacher she was deaf, and this was signalled by her use of hearing aids. Like many invisible disabilities, being deaf can be hard to quantify as initially there are few visual cues.

If your deafness is caused by a single event – for example, your eardrum being perforated, the first signs can be immediate. However, most people realise more slowly that they are not hearing at the same level as those around them. This was my experience too, and this is what I will explore in this chapter. I can't remember what my very first signs were; the moments build over time and then all of a sudden you realise it is right there staring at you in the face.

The NHS website says the first signs of hearing loss include:

- difficulty hearing other people clearly and misunderstanding what they say, especially in noisy places
- asking people to repeat themselves
- listening to music or watching TV with the volume higher than other people need
- difficulty hearing on the phone
- finding it hard to keep up with a conversation
- feeling tired or stressed from having to concentrate while listening[10]

So basically the main sign of hearing loss is that you can't hear very well. Seems pretty obvious, doesn't it? Seriously, though, it is important to have these symptoms written down in a list, as seeing them all together can create a lightbulb moment. If you're having problems with one of the things on this list, you could put this down to something else, but the whole list? I could tick off everything on this list of symptoms, but initially

I put it all down to other factors. I thought I had difficulty understanding people in noisy places because the places were loud and people weren't talking loudly and clearly enough – that's right, it's not me, it's you. A psychologist would say, 'Sam, why are you blaming others rather than looking inside yourself?' – or looking inside my ear, in this case. I also put asking people to repeat themselves down to noisy places, quiet talkers or unusual accents. That's right, I even blamed buildings and 'foreign people' for my hearing loss – I sound like a politician. Sorry. I reasoned that I listened to TV and music extra-loud because I like to be fully immersed in the sound because I'm a theatrical person, which is also true.

I never noticed that I had difficulty hearing on the phone because I didn't like speaking to new people on the phone so I just avoided it. I wonder why! I definitely found it hard to keep up with some conversations, but reasoned this was because I was usually playing Candy Crush or checking Instagram at the same time. Yes, let's blame technology too – that's the reason I didn't book a hearing test. I was definitely concentrating hard on listening, which made me tired and stressed, but I just believed that I was tired and stressed generally . . . which was fine because that meant I was allowed to book myself a spa day and eat some cake to treat myself and relax.

Looking back, I can see so many signs that I was struggling in a hearing world, but at the time it was easy to blame them on something or someone else. When I was younger, I wrote my sister's name on my bedroom wall in crayon, then lied to my parents and said my little sister had written it. The only problem was, my little sister was a baby at the time. I guess I've always been good at making excuses.

But I wasn't the only one. Activist Charlotte Hyde recalls: 'I had no clue I was deaf until I was diagnosed. I thought everyone put the subtitles on the telly, that lyric booklets in CDs existed because song lyrics were difficult to hear for everyone, and that struggling with my balance was normal.'

I struggled with my balance too as I have one-sided deafness. For years I saw a physiotherapist who gave me exercises for my weak ankle, which I had blamed as the reason I was always falling over on my right-hand side. I'd like to formally apologise to my ankle for calling her weak and blaming her for something she didn't do. To this day, no one has officially told me that my balance issues are down to my one-sided deafness, but today I never fall over when I'm wearing my hearing aid. To me that is proof. You might also rely on other people telling you that you have a problem and that you should seek help. It is a sentiment I can relate to. I was waiting on someone else to tell me I needed to get my hearing checked, whether this was a health professional or family/friend. I wasn't ready to deal with the issue myself.

You might make excuses, like I did, or you might not even know what being deaf actually means. Keighley Miles, from Essex-based youth group Families of Deaf Children, says: 'Looking back, I remember saying to a friend "I don't know what they're saying on the TV, so I make up my own stories in my head – do you?" So I suppose that was a major sign, but I didn't know that I was deaf. I thought I was just weird/different.'

How would you know that this was a sign of deafness if no one had ever told you?

As I have mentioned, it takes on average ten years for someone to notice the signs of hearing loss and deafness and do something about them. It's a shocking statistic, but one I can relate to. Please don't make the same mistake I did: if you think you're experiencing any of the signs of deafness listed above, then please book a hearing test as soon as possible. The sooner you discover you are deaf, the sooner you can get support, whether this means having hearing aids fitted, starting to learn BSL, or finding your local deaf community.

I think I have noticed the signs – what now?

The next step is to complete a hearing test. You can get a hearing test through the NHS by going to your GP, who will refer you. You can also get a hearing test from a private audiologist. To find your nearest registered audiologist, go to the British Society of Hearing Aid Audiologists website (www. BSHAA.org). High-street chemist Boots also does hearing tests, as does Amplifon, which has branches across the country. Usually the hearing test is free and the audiologist will advise you about which hearing aid might work for you, if any. A hearing test is like an eye test: the test may cost a minimal amount, then it's the glasses or the hearing aid that you pay for. If you can't afford to buy your own hearing aids then you can get them on the NHS; however, you might have to wait several months for an appointment. It is also worth noting that hearing aids available on the NHS are not always as advanced as hearing aids available in the private sector.

RNID also have a handy hearing test on their website (www. rnid.org.uk). If you're worried about going to your GP or an audiologist, you can use this online test to give you an indication of whether a hearing test might be a good next step.

The first time I noticed I hadn't heard something

I want to tell you about the first time I noticed that I didn't hear something, and someone else did. It was something important too. I was on a boat at a comedy gig – yes, you can have comedy anywhere, even on a boat. I was MCing the evening, which basically means that I kicked off the night, welcomed the audience, did some jokes and audience chat, introduced each act on stage and wrapped up at the end. I got there nice and early because I'm a professional and because I hadn't performed there before and I wanted to scope the venue out: by that I mean I wanted to find out where the toilets were. I need to know how close the toilets are in all situations. I know what you're thinking – and yes, I am super fun to be around. It's not just that I like to pee a lot (which I do), but the toilets can be a sanctuary for deaf people like me, especially when the noise gets too loud or listening gets too tiring.

There were also some brilliant comedians on the bill that night, so I wanted to do a great job to impress my peers. The rather large boat was on the Thames in London. The boat was split into several bar areas and a comedy area, which did not bode well from a sound perspective. The comedy area was its own closed-off room (phew, no bar noises) that could seat about 200 audience members, but that night it was only half full as it was a Thursday rather than a weekend show. Weekday shows tend to be full of drunk City workers wanting a laugh, to take off their ties (such rebels) and drink several pints of vodka. This meant there was lots of empty space for sound to echo around. Did you know that bodies absorb sound? It's true – next time you're in a loud environment, try using your partner's body to muffle the sound by putting your face to their back or chest. It works – plus, you usually get a hug out of it.

The back of the stage had a vivid red velvet curtain across it, separating the performance/audience area from the backstage area. Alas, velvet helps but does not block out all sound, meaning only a thin piece of material separated us comedians from our uninterested public. As the crowd started to file in, I noticed that we were so close we could smell them – and definitely hear them.

Backstage, the comics were all a bit nervous: it was a new material night, so some of the jokes had never been said aloud before. It's rare for a brand-new joke to get a wonderful response on its first outing, as the wording and delivery usually take a certain amount of tweaking. However, all comedians still live in hope that golden nuggets will trickle out of our brains and be perfectly honed, well-structured jokes that need no work whatsoever . . . a lot like the first draft of a book. Ah, we can but dream. As we waited behind our velvet screen, anxiously rewriting our jokes, the audience were making it known they existed by shedding coats, talking loudly, scraping chairs and clinking glasses. The sound and lighting technician was also playing loud, upbeat music to create a lively comedy atmosphere, and I happened to be sitting under the speaker. As you can probably guess, this wasn't the ideal environment for someone who is deaf, but of course at the time I hadn't yet realised that I was deaf – or why I felt so stressed every time I was at work. I thought all comedians felt that way. To be honest, it's a pretty stress-inducing job. That night the noise was so loud that my tinnitus flared up, but at the time I didn't know what that was either.

Then it happened.

The first time I noticed that I didn't hear something and someone else did.

It was a small moment, but it had a huge impact on my life. It set off a chain of events that led me to writing this book. I guess it's like the film adaptation of *Lemony Snicket's Series of Unfortunate Events* – but without a voiceover by Jude Law (do you think he'd do the audiobook?) and without Jim Carrey's amazing dinosaur impression (before he went off films and got really into art). Don't worry if you haven't seen it; that description won't spoil it for you.

That night also ended up being a series of rather *fortunate* events! So let's imagine this important moment in slow motion and with sad, yet dramatic, *X-Factor* back-story music over the top – you know, how deafness is usually portrayed on screen, to make it feel really important. Picture the scene: I was standing facing the technician (the person who's in charge of lighting and sound) and she said something to me. Over the music and the sounds of the audience, I couldn't hear anything she said – and I mean I couldn't even make out a single word. I concentrated hard as I tried to lip-read or hear some semblance of a sentence, but I got nothing. Inside I could feel myself shrugging and thinking, 'This woman is talking too quietly. Doesn't she realise she needs to speak loudly over all the noise?' Then I turned to see another comedian standing next to me. He smiled and replied to the technician as if it was the most natural thing in the world. That was it – the first time I didn't hear something someone else did. It sounds so small and uneventful, but I remember it vividly, and it knocked the wind out of me. Not being able to hear at that moment was particularly annoying, as the technician had been telling me she was about to announce my name. A second later, she was saying my name in a microphone to a quietening crowd and pushing me through the thin curtain on stage to be funny.

So that was my first time. Then I immediately went to the doctors to get a hearing test, right?! Wrong. It was at least a year before I did that, and when I did, it wasn't because of mishearing something. It was because I thought I had something living in my ear – true story, which I will tell later (see p. 143).

Chapter 4

What to expect at a hearing test

In my experience, most people go for a hearing test when they think they have a problem, rather than having an annual hearing check. You know, it's like when you wait until the last possible moment to finish that presentation rather than doing it in advance and avoiding all the added stress. I think regular hearing tests are as important as regular eye tests and dentist appointments.

Sorry, I just had to pause a moment to call my dentist, who said I am no longer registered with them as they haven't seen me for a few years. They assumed I'd moved house. Oops. Anyway, do as I say, not as I do . . .

Audiologist Adam Chell agrees with me about hearing tests: 'Everybody should have a fifteen-minute hearing screen at least every three years.'

So why doesn't this happen? Why isn't this the norm? Amplifon audiologist Jane Noble advises: 'Generally, people aged sixty and older should have a baseline hearing test and get their hearing checked every few years to rule out age-related hearing loss. People working in noisy occupations, even if they're younger than sixty, should consider having a hearing screen every few years to ensure the noise isn't affecting their hearing.' RNID chief exec Mark Atkinson agrees with the audiologists: 'At RNID, we want everyone to look after their hearing the way they look after their eyes or their teeth.'

So why aren't we listening to the experts?

Well, there seems to be a real stigma around hearing loss and deafness, connected to the idea of getting old before your time – but for some reason there isn't the same stigma around eye tests and glasses. I am trying my best to be a young(ish), hip-young-thing example of a hearing-aid wearer, but it's obviously not enough. Maybe we need designer hearing aids just like we have designer glasses frames? Or do we need more adverts on TV to normalise getting hearing aids and to let people see them in all their glory, like those dental hygiene adverts for whitening toothpaste?

Perhaps you're scared of what might happen during a hearing test. Will you have to take off all your clothes, like you do for an MRI scan? Will someone shout at you until you hear them properly? Or will you be given a grey wig and have boiled sweets sewn into your pockets? Thankfully, none of the above are part of a standard hearing test, but in case you were wondering what actually happens, I have described this mysterious experience below.

Newborn hearing test

The newborn hearing test was rolled out widely in 1992. A baby's hearing can be tested from as young as four weeks old and up to three months. It does not hurt the baby in any way. During a newborn hearing test, a small earpiece is put into the baby's ear that plays soft clicking noises. Repeat tests may be done with head sensors if the first test is inconclusive. Using this test, most cases of deafness in newborns should be picked up straight away. If the test shows that your child has full hearing but you see symptoms that make you think otherwise – perhaps your baby doesn't respond to loud noises, or turn when they hear your voice – please persist and take them to see a health visitor or GP. As deaf actor Sophie Stone says, 'doctors don't know everything', and a parent/guardian or teacher who spends time with children may be the first to notice any signs of deafness.

Is the newborn hearing test necessary? Well, the NHS website states that: '1 to 2 babies in every 1,000 are born with permanent hearing loss in one or both ears. This increases to about 1 in every 100 babies who have spent more than 48 hours in intensive care. Most of these babies are born into families with no history of permanent hearing loss.' So yes, the newborn hearing test is very important.

Adult hearing tests

There are two types of adult hearing test: a short one and a longer one. Audiologist Adam Chell explains, 'You have your ears looked in and listen to some beeps and whistles to measure the quietest sound you can hear. This may take fifteen minutes, and requires very little knowledge or experience to conduct. Alternatively, you can have an assessment that lasts over two hours. The purpose of this assessment is to determine your hearing profile.' (A hearing profile is an in-depth look at your hearing loss, levels, pitches and how your hearing loss might affect you in noisy surroundings.)

I have had both types of hearing test. The shorter option found out that I had some hearing loss, while the second test was more extensive, discovering more specific aspects of my hearing loss and determining what tools might be available to me, including hearing aids.

Amplifon Audiologist Jane Noble goes into a little more detail:

> The hearing assessment begins with otoscopy, where your audiologist will look inside your ear and examine the health of your ear canals and eardrums. The next part of the assessment usually involves pure-tone audiometry, which includes listening to tones at different pitches and volumes, then speech testing where your audiologist looks at your speech recognition in quiet and in noise, which shows how you might get on with hearing aids. Your audiologist will then take some time to go through the results and look at the next steps with you.

(For those who don't know, 'speech recognition in quiet and in noise' involves listening to someone talking over the top of different levels of background noise.)

Interestingly, I don't remember ever having a hearing test until *the* test during that I found out I had hearing loss – and yes, 'hearing loss' was the phrase used by the audiologist. *The* test took place when I was twenty-nine. It's shocking to think that I went almost three decades without any sort of hearing test.

When I was around seven I had grommets inserted in my ears – a procedure to relieve glue ear. I didn't have a hearing test before this; the doctor simply looked in my ears and determined that the symptoms my parents had noticed were down to glue ear. Glue ear is where the empty middle part of the ear canal fills up with fluid.[11] It's more common in children, but adults can sometimes get it too. It can cause temporary hearing loss, but it usually clears up within a few months.

Grommets are small tubes that are inserted surgically to drain fluid from the ear. I'm ashamed to say I was thirty years old when I discovered this. I had always imagined that grommets were small hearing aids that had been inserted into my ears to help me hear. As I child I remember going to the doctor, who reached into my ear with tweezers to remove one of the grommets, which had fallen out of place and was no longer needed. He showed me the grommet. It looked like a small white plastic tube, but that still didn't stop me thinking it was a hearing aid.

What is a hearing test like?

So we have heard what a hearing test is like from the people who conduct them, but what is one like for someone going through the process? Interior designer Micaela Sharp remembers:

> I completed a hearing test which involved clicking a button when you heard a bleep. Starting on my healthier side, perhaps quite cruelly, I eagerly clicked along. When the time came to listen with my damaged ear, I quickly realised that I couldn't hear any bleeps, and had to hold back tears. I was expecting to be prescribed a solution – some ear drops, perhaps, and to return to full hearing, but the doctor told me that I had permanently lost quite a lot of range on one side and I needed a hearing aid.

In contrast, my realisation of my hearing loss didn't come until after the test. You see, I practise a lot of self-belief, so of course

I thought I had nailed the hearing test and had 20/20 hearing (which isn't a thing).

Looking back on *the* hearing test, it's all a bit of a blur, mainly due to my shock. I had been referred by my GP and thought that the test was merely a formality to double-check my hearing, so I felt very blasé about it. I arrived in Stratford in London at a small, nondescript grey building. I walked through the glass double doors and panicked immediately. This was a hearing test centre – would the people who worked here be deaf? Would I have to use sign language? I didn't know any sign language, and suddenly felt very foolish and unprepared. I walked up to reception and smiled, which seemed the safest option. The receptionist said something like, 'Here for a hearing test?' I sighed with relief, answered, and was directed into a waiting room.

I had heard about a hearing test called 'a beep test'. I wasn't entirely sure what that meant, but I wasn't too nervous – after all, my hearing was fine. I used to tell a joke about this test: 'The only beep test I'd done previously was the one where you run between the cones at school. So I turned up in full Lycra. There was an eighty-year-old man in the waiting room and I thought, "He's going to struggle."'

It wasn't quite like that, but I was immediately struck by the other people in the waiting room. They all had grey hair and were much older than me. I was brought into a room that was acoustically padded. The sound in the room is worth mentioning, because if you have never been in a sound studio before, you will notice the difference. There is an absence of background noise, and the air feels slightly more oppressive, due to the cushioning of the sound. Then I was directed to a small booth with a chair inside, a lot like a toilet cubicle with a window. You may be asked to sit in front of a fan-shaped desktop machine instead of a booth. The audiologist placed headphones over my ears and told me to listen out for beeps and to try to ignore any white noise I might hear. You are either given a small clicking device to press, like the ones TV weather presenters use (if you are in a booth), or you're told to say something out loud like 'yes' (if you are sitting at a desk) when you hear a beep. The process will be repeated with the headphones in different positions – for example, the headphone over your left ear but off your right. The audiologist might even change the set of headphones for a pair that have one headphone and one flat panel that sits behind your ear. The process will then be repeated but, instead of beeps, there will be other sounds and/or voices talking over background noise, and you will have to click when you hear a sound and repeat out loud any words you hear. Throughout this process you will be doing your serious concentration face and squinting and straining to hear, so it will be very tiring. It's definitely worth bringing a sugary snack/beverage to consume afterwards so you have the energy to get yourself home. For competitive readers (I'm very competitive), it's worth pointing out that the beeps happen randomly and can be controlled by the audiologist, so there is no cheating or learning the sequence and then clicking from memory. Sorry! I don't know why I wanted to cheat at my hearing test, as it was for my own benefit, but nevertheless the temptation was there. If you have tinnitus, it's worth telling your audiologist this, as the beeping can sound like certain types of tinnitus. Or it can even bring on your tinnitus, which can make things confusing. The audiologist may be able to change the pitch of beep to help with this. Quite often I would click after hearing a phantom beep, which had probably been caused by my tinnitus.

For my hearing test I was in a sound booth (the toilet cubicle option). Having had hearing tests at a desk and at a booth, I prefer the booth, as I can focus on the test rather than any external stimuli. I know it was a booth because I distinctly remember finishing the test and strutting out of it like the sort of smug person who says they don't really have to study for exams. I truly thought I had aced the hearing test. I was waiting for the audiologist to tell me that I had achieved the highest ever hearing test score and start engraving my name on some sort of champions board. But this didn't happen.

After the test I sat down opposite the audiologist. They didn't immediately give me a diagnosis. Instead they brought up my hearing graphs for each ear and showed me what 'normal' hearing looked like and, by contrast, what my graphs looked like. At this point I remember thinking, 'Oh right, I have some hearing loss – interesting.' However, when I heard him say, 'You have hearing loss in both ears but it is significant enough on one side that we would advise you to use a hearing aid', my stomach dropped. It was a 'jaw-on-the-floor, rabbit-in-the-headlights' moment. It was the scary words 'hearing aid' that really hit home, with all their stereotypes and connotations, which felt so far removed from me and my life. I was told I would be booked in for a hearing-aid fitting, given some leaflets and sent on my way. I wandered back to Stratford train station in a daze. I remember glancing at the leaflets, which showed a couple with white hair looking happy, as if they were newly retired and moving to their new countryside getaway. The only person on the leaflets who looked anything like me was the nurse who was helping the newly retired people.

As I got closer to the station the reality of what I had been told hit me and I felt the need to cry – well, not cry, but sob like a toddler. As I'm British, I didn't want to sob on the street, so I managed to find a quiet corner – which happened to be the bicycle storage shelter of Westfield Stratford Shopping Centre. Surrounded by bikes locked to metal bars, I let the tears come and called my mum. I'm surprised my mum managed to understand anything I said in that phone call, but mums always have a way, don't they?

'I know it is a shock, but it's fine. I have hearing aids too,' said my Mum.

'Yeah, but you're sixty and I'm almost thirty, Mum.'

Later on, I would be very glad that I had someone in my life who also wore hearing aids and understood what that meant. (Also please don't tell my mum I put her age in this book – she will kill me.)

Over time, I would come to love my hearing aid and deafness, and it would lead to some of the best moments/achievements in my life (read more about this in Chapter 20), but that after-noon in the bike shed at Westfield Shopping Centre Stratford I couldn't see any of that, so I carried on sobbing. In fact, I sobbed so much that when a woman walked in, presumably to retrieve her bike, she made eye contact with me and slowly backed away. Maybe she thought I had a puncture or I really, really cared about sustainable transport.

Want a hearing test?

To reiterate, RNID have an online hearing test for anyone who wants to check their hearing and get an idea of whether they might need to see an audiologist. It takes about three minutes and will tell you what next steps you need to take. To take the test, go to rnid.org.uk.

If you want to see an audiologist for a hearing test you can either book an appointment with your GP, who will refer you, or you can book a private hearing test with a provider like Boots, Specsavers, Amplifon or an independent local audiologist.

If you're worried about what to expect or what type of test you might have, just ask the receptionist about the test when you book, or check out the provider's website, which should have all the information you need.

Chapter 5
Hearing aids

The most important thing to note is that hearing aids do not 'reverse' hearing loss. Nor do they help you to hear 'normally'. Author Jaipreet Virdi describes them 'as one of the many tools that will enable [users] to navigate through the hearing world'.[12]

I am sure we have all seen those videos doing the rounds on the internet showing a baby or young person having their hearing aids switched on for the first time, when a look of wonder crosses their face and their parents weep with joy. In real life, having a hearing aid switched on for the first time is overwhelming. It's loud and emotional, yes, but not necessarily because the person can suddenly hear everything they have always wanted to. It's emotional because there's a lot of sound hitting you all at once and your brain hasn't had time to catch up. But once your brain has had time to catch up (which can take a few weeks), hearing aids can be an amazing tool to help you in day-to-day life – if you choose to use them.

What are hearing aids, and why might you need them?

Audiologist Adam Chell says:

> Hearing aids are an investment in your future self. By getting a hearing aid today instead of in ten years' time, you are much

more likely to perform well with it. Your dexterity, brain plasticity and muscle memory all help you to get on with a hearing aid. By adopting one early when perhaps you don't need it as much, you can ensure that when you really need it in later life, you are practised and prepared.

That being said, using hearing aids is a personal choice. Many deaf people decide not to use them and are living awesome, fulfilling lives. In addition, hearing aids don't work for all kinds of deafness, so telling someone they should get hearing aids if they are deaf or have hearing loss isn't always useful. There are different types of hearing aids for different deaf experiences, and Amplifon audiologist Jane Noble explains these here:

> Hearing aids come in many different styles. The most common styles are the following:
>
> - **Behind-the-ear (BTE):** hearing aids which sit behind the ear with tubing that routes the sound to the ear.
> - **Receiver-in-the-ear (RITE):** Like a BTE, the bulk of the hearing aid sits behind the ear, with a thin wire (not tubing) that connects the hearing aid to a speaker sitting inside the ear.
> - **In-the-ear (ITE):** Hearing aids that sit completely in your ear, typically customised to fit in your ear. In-the-ear styles include small, invisible-in-the-canal (IIC), completely-in-the-canal (CIC), larger in-the-canal (ITC) and in-the-ear (ITE) types.

I have used ITEs in the past. They are very discreet, but I found that, as I still have some residual hearing, they were blocking up my ear canal too much. I also kept losing my ITE hearing aid as I would take it out and leave it in random places in the house and forget where I had left it – but that's probably a me problem.

I now use a RITE hearing aid, which works really well for me. It lets sounds into my ear and improves on the sounds I might miss by amplifying them. I still sometimes leave it in random places around the house, but at least when I do this it's larger and easier to spot. I have a silver Phonak Audeo hearing aid and a pink Widex one from Amplifon. (Full disclosure: these hearing aids were very kindly gifted to me, as I am a deaf influencer these days. I love them both. I prefer the sound quality with the Phonak hearing aid, but I love that the Widex one is bright pink!)

What type of hearing aid is right for you?

Jane Noble explains how your audiologist should approach this: 'We take time discussing each style and together find something that fits your needs and hearing levels, as not every hearing aid is suitable for everyone.' It can be a bit of a process to find the right aid for you and what you need: it's kind of like finding the perfect cut of jeans . . . but slightly more important, depending on how trouser-obsessed you are, of course.

Other types of hearing aid, as listed on the NHS website, are:

- **Body-worn hearing aids:** 'Body-worn hearing aids are made up of a small box connected to earphones. The box can be clipped to your clothes or put inside a pocket. This type of hearing aid may be best if you have severe hearing loss and need a powerful hearing aid, or if you find the controls on smaller hearing aids tricky to use.'

- **CROS** and **BiCROS hearing aids:** 'CROS and BiCROS hearing aids can help if you've lost hearing in one ear. They come as a pair. The hearing aid in the ear with hearing loss picks up sound and sends it to a hearing aid in your good ear. This can be done wirelessly or through a wire around the back of your neck.'[13]

But how do they work? The Boots website – yes, you can get hearing aids from Boots – explains:

A hearing aid is usually made up of three main components:

- The microphone picks up sounds from the environment and transmits them to the processor.
- The processor analyses the sounds and converts them into electrical signals.
- The loudspeaker or receiver transmits these signals to your ear, where it's released as sound so you can hear and understand it.

Hearing aids don't just make everything louder: they amplify the sounds that you need for communication and reduce the disruptive sounds you don't want.[14]

Audiologist and founder of hearing-aid jewellery company Little Auricles Rita Kairouz says: 'Hearing aids are amazing, but they don't work miracles. They help deaf and hard of hearing people access sound, but visual cues are still extremely important.'

Many deaf people, including me, use hearing aids alongside lip-reading and BSL as well as other tools.

Hearing aids are constantly advancing, just like any other technology. Amplifon audiologist Jane Noble explains that: 'Audiology is heavily reliant on equipment and technology which is always changing and improving, allowing audiologists to make real changes in lives. Most newer hearing aids can directly connect with mobile phones and tablets.' My hearing aid connects to my phone, which is one of the things people are always most impressed by. When I give talks to groups of children about deafness (one of my favourite things to do), I always say that when my mum tells me off I listen to Beyoncé through my hearing aid so I can't hear her. Kids seem to like the idea of that! I have been known to listen (via my hearing aid) to music or podcasts during boring talks I have had to sit through, and it means I can watch TikTok and Instagram videos on loud when I'm on public transport without annoying anyone, as the sound comes through my hearing aid. I can also answer my phone with my hearing aid and speak to someone, just like you would with a Bluetooth headset. However, my sixty-something-year-old mum has the same capability with her hearing aids and constantly wanders away from her phone during a call, which makes the sound cut out – so that is something to be aware of!

It is not just Bluetooth capabilities that help to stream sound. Jane Noble says: 'Connection to an app gives you the added advantage of having your smartphone function as a remote control, allowing you to tweak the volume and equalisation.' Some hearing aids can connect to apps, which allow them to translate different languages! That's actually where the idea for my children's book *Harriet Versus the Galaxy* (available in all good bookshops) came from. In the book, Harriet's hearing aid translates alien languages and, with her gran (who doesn't have a hearing aid), she protects the Earth from aliens . . . as you do.

Even tech giant Apple is getting involved, with their Conversation Boost setting for AirPods:

> Conversation Boost for AirPods Pro helps you better hear conversations in crowded or noisy environments. Through computational audio and beamforming microphones, Conversation Boost focuses AirPods Pro on the voice of the person directly in front of you, making it easier to distinguish speech and follow along in face-to-face conversations.[15]

More and more modern hearing aids are also rechargeable. They come with a charging port that you plug them into at night, just like you charge your phone. This means that there's no need to purchase small batteries to power your hearing aids, which was always the case before. My first hearing aid used small batteries that were very fiddly and had tiny stickers on them that you had to remove before fitting the battery. One unexpected side effect of using these batteries was that I was constantly finding bright yellow hearing-aid battery stickers all over my house and clothes. They're like glitter: you keep finding them for years afterwards.

When I spoke to audiologist Adam Chell about the future of hearing aids he was very excited, and his enthusiasm was contagious:

> Technology is improving at an exponential rate. Big tech like Apple is getting behind hearing health, and global

manufacturers are getting more daring with their designs and features. At the time of writing we already have hearing aids that are waterproof, have Bluetooth, take phone calls, monitor your heart rate, count the steps you walk, or even detect if you have fallen over and automatically text an emergency contact with your exact location. It's just amazing. In the future, hearing aids may be able to measure your hydration levels, and even monitor changes in your cognitive function for diseases like dementia and Alzheimer's.

It is pretty incredible that your hearing aid could save your life in the future by notifying an emergency contact that you are in peril. The possibilities are exciting. Perhaps one day everyone will wear a hearing device, using it as a phone and monitoring system even if they aren't deaf. I am, however, slightly less excited about monitoring my step count and hydration levels. I don't feel like I need any more reminders that I don't walk enough or drink enough water!

Cochlear implants

So what are cochlear implants? They are an aid for hearing, introduced in the 1970s but not usually considered a 'hearing aid' in the general sense, as they are classified as an implant. In 2022 one contestant on the reality show *Love Island*, Tasha Ghouri, had a cochlear implant, which seemed to cause a lot of confusion on social media. So let's clear up this confusion, on behalf of reality-TV contestants everywhere.

The RNID website says:

Cochlear implants have several different parts, some of which are internal (cannot be seen) and some of which are external (worn on the body).

- The internal part consists of a receiver with a magnet that is fitted under the skin behind the ear, plus electrodes inserted into the cochlea.
- The external part consists of a microphone and sound processor with a transmitter coil. Sound is picked up by the microphone in the cochlear implant and processed into electrical signals that are passed to the transmitter coil.

The transmitter coil sends signals, by radio wave, through the skin to the implanted receiver. The receiver sends the signals down the wire to the electrodes in the cochlea. When the electrodes receive the signal, a tiny electric current stimulates the auditory nerve to provide a sensation of hearing.[16]

RNID also explains that 'cochlear implants provide a sensation of hearing to those who have severe to profound deafness. This means that they may be able to hear some sounds, but not all that make up human speech.'

What's it actually like to get a cochlear implant, though? RNID advocacy officer Annie Harris describes her experience:

I decided to get a cochlear implant, and had the operation in January 2005, four months into my first year at uni. I couldn't hear anything for a month, and it was very painful as I developed an infection. When I had it switched on, the sounds were very weird, and distorting – like robotic beats for every sound. It felt like being underwater. I had to persevere, and eventually sounds became more familiar over time.

Thankfully, the experience did get better for Annie:

It's been worth it in the long term, because now I can enjoy listening to music, and one-to-one conversations with my husband and family. I couldn't live without my implant now. But I wish that people realised that cochlear implants don't mean that we are suddenly able to hear. People see me speaking clearly and automatically presume I can hear too.

As Annie mentioned, cochlear implants are inserted under general anaesthetic during an operation. Some deaf people choose not to have them, even if an audiologist believes they may benefit the person. Actor Sophie Stone reveals: 'Today I was (again) offered a cochlear implant. I proudly stated that I'm happy just the way I am. The nurse replied, "I respect that." The first time I felt heard in an audiology room – the irony.'

While some people choose not to have a cochlear implant, others can't get the implants they need – and want. Keighley Miles, who runs the Families of Deaf Children community group, explains: 'I only have one cochlear implant, even though I'm profoundly deaf in both ears. I had it as an adult and the NHS only funds one for adults.' As of 2022, it is still the case that the NHS only funds one cochlear implant, unless you are a deafblind adult or have other sensory needs. However, this is different for children, who are able to have two cochlear implants via the NHS.

In 2019 the BBC reported that 'the total cost of a cochlear implant for one ear, including the surgery, is £22,919, and for two ears it is £37,904'.[17] Yes, they are pricey, but can you put a price on helping someone hear so they face fewer accessibility barriers?

Bone-anchored hearing aids (BAHAs)

The NHS website explains:

> A bone-anchored hearing aid (BAHA) may be an option if you have hearing loss caused by sound being unable to reach your inner ear. This type of hearing aid is attached to your skull during a minor operation. It picks up sound and sends it to the inner ear by vibrating the bones near your ear. It can be clipped on and off – for example, it's removed at night and when you swim or take a shower. Some newer types are held on to the head with magnets instead of a connector through the skin.[18]

Do hearing aids whistle?

I will let audiologist Adam Chell answer this one:

> Hearing aids shouldn't whistle when they are in your ear. If they are whistling while you are wearing them, it's likely to be one of three things:
>
> 1) Excessive ear wax.
> 2) Not inserted correctly.

3) Not fitting correctly – e.g. dome too small or vents too large.

Hearing aids usually whistle a bit when outside the ear, though, and this is completely normal. If you are having persistent whistling, go back to your audiologist.

Amplifon audiologist Jane Noble agrees: 'Feedback is normal as you put in your hearing aids, but if it continues when the hearing aids are in, you should seek help from your audiologist.'

I am always shocked by how many people ask me this question. Even an experienced radio producer recently asked me if my hearing aid would whistle and interfere with equipment when I was in the radio studio, about to go on air! The answer is no, and I have proven this many times while talking on the phone on the radio, on FaceTime/Zoom on the radio, and in the studio. So don't worry, my hearing aid won't affect your enjoyment of Lady Gaga's latest track.

Are hearing aids any good, though?

Well, I would say that mine is great. It's particularly helpful in noisy environments like restaurants or bars, by dulling background noise, and it reminded me that I had been missing certain sounds. I had forgotten that I could hear birdsong from my back garden, and my hearing aid helped me get back that beautiful sound.

The tech is getting better and better, as I mentioned earlier and as Mark Atkinson, RNID chief exec, reveals: 'Technology has moved on enormously from when RNID was started – the days of big clunky hearing aids are in the past. All hearing aids available on the NHS or privately are digital, which means they are prescription-fitted to your individual needs.' So if it's clunky, whistley technology that you're worried about, then you have no need to fear.

Mark goes on to say:

> Hearing loss can cause isolation and can increase the risk of dementia by up to five times, but evidence suggests that hearing aids may reduce these risks. There is a growing body of research that demonstrates the strong benefits of people taking action as early as possible if they have concerns about their hearing, by getting their hearing checked and wearing hearing aids if they need to.

So if wearing hearing aids could reduce the risk of feeling isolated – which it has definitely done for me – and reduce the risk of dementia, then it doesn't sound like a bad thing. However, I respect people's right to choose not to wear one and to be happy just as they are, as Sophie Stone said. I would like to see more research into the mental health and physical health benefits of hearing aids.

Interior designer Micaela Sharp says: 'I have a hearing aid. I loved using it at first, particularly the background noise-cancelling function when I was out for dinner. That was a game-changer! Finally I could sit at a table with someone on my bad ear side and still communicate fully.' However, now she rarely wears hers. Annie Harris, RNID advocacy officer, agrees: 'Growing up, I had two hearing aids. Unfortunately, in 2017, my hearing declined rapidly in my left ear so I rarely wear a hearing aid in that ear now.'

Many people start off well with hearing aids, then resist them further down the line. This may be due to lifestyle, stigma or other personal choices, but I would advise you to persist if they support your day-to-day life.

Most hearing-aid providers will offer a free trial of a hearing aid. I would suggest that, even if you're not sure it's worth trying a hearing aid. You might be pleasantly surprised!

How much do hearing aids cost?

Hearing aids are currently free on the NHS. The NHS website explains that when you buy a hearing aid privately, 'You can pay anything from £500 to £3,500 or more for a single hearing aid.' I know – now you're more impressed that I am a deaf influencer, hey? I might not get free holidays or do yoga poses in front of incredible vistas, but I'm lucky enough to get top-of-the-range hearing aids, which I use every day.

If cost is a worry for you, Amplifon audiologist Jane Noble advises: 'Hearing aids are available at multiple price points to fit most needs, and most retailers will have finance options available, helping you spread out the cost into easy and affordable payments.'

Hearing assistive devices, like a microphone worn around a speaker's neck (see p. 131), can also be expensive but, depending on your personal situation, you may be able to apply for a grant to pay for those.

A history of hearing aids

'Skin of serpent boiled in wine, fat of fox's lungs, egg yolks and goose grease' were all on the list of ingredients for an ear ointment to 'cure' deafness, explains Jaipreet Virdi in her book *Hearing Happiness: Deafness Cures in History*.[19] It definitely has a 'witches from *Macbeth*' vibe, as lists go – I encourage you to read the list out loud in your best witchy voice. Jaipreet goes on to describe her research into 'medical textbooks listing descriptions of experiments using burning caustics, blistering, setons, or hammering deaf children's skulls' to 'cure' deafness. As we know today, there is no cure for being deaf, because deafness is not a disease. Not only would these methods not have worked, but they also sound like actual methods of torture (FYI, caustics are corrosive substances that cause particularly bad burns, and a seton is a stitch that goes through the skin and is left protruding to encourage drainage). Before hearing aids, these were the only options available! Thank God we don't live in a bygone era – although I did once play a wench in a comedy show called *Sunny D* on BBC3, and I have to say the look suited me.

In the early 1600s, before hearing aids, came hearing trumpets: large metal trumpets that you'd hold to your ear, making you look a lot like a human gramophone. I don't think high-street retailer Boots was around in the 1600s, but their website explains hearing trumpets:

> In the 17th century, it took a big, cumbersome device to help people with hearing loss. Funnel-shaped hearing trumpets amplified sounds by 20–30 dB. While they were large and not very portable, they were effective! It was the

invention of the telephone in the 19th century that paved the way for the development of the electric hearing aid. But at the time, telephone technology was still too cumbersome.

In the mid-1800s there was an invention called the 'aural vibrator', which sounds rather fun: its aim was to use vibrations to break up any blockages in your ear. But as soon as ear trumpets were on the scene, so was people's desire to hide them or make them seem invisible – an attitude that continues today. 'Urns, fans, thrones, headbands and walking canes contained cleverly obscured ear trumpets'[20] – now, come on, don't tell me you've never wanted your own throne!

Howard Alexander writes in *The New York Times*:

The earliest hearing aid was simplicity itself, and is still in use: a cupped hand behind the ear. But today's technology has made hearing aids much less obtrusive and much more helpful . . . In 1913 Siemens became one of the first companies to offer electronically amplified hearing aids. These early units were large and not very portable – about the size of a tall cigar box – but they had a speaker that fit into the ear . . . Until the early 1990s, most hearing aids were analogue and consisted of a microphone, an amplifier and a speaker (transducer). But with the availability of miniature computer components, as well as the audio-processing technology found in CD and DVD players, the digital hearing aid was born.[21]

Most hearing aids today are digital, and these advances mean we have much more control over how we hear sound, using particular hearing-aid settings. Howard Alexander goes on to explain:

> What these settings do is adjust the equalisation, volume and signal-processing functions. If you cannot hear high frequencies well but love chamber music, the appropriate setting would emphasise the high frequencies (for the violins) and give you a moderate increase in volume. Lunch with the boss would require an emphasis on the middle range (for the human voice), a decrease in the high frequencies and some form of extraneous noise reduction.[22]

Will hearing aids make my hearing worse?

No – they're not like glasses, which your eyes can become reliant on and so stop trying. God, eyes are lazy! Adam Chell explains: 'Hearing aids, if prescribed appropriately, should not accelerate the rate of hearing deterioration.' Whether your hearing will get worse generally is another matter. It is important to protect your hearing by limiting your exposure to loud sounds, even when you have assistive devices like hearing aids.

Persevering with hearing aids

So you've been given a hearing aid or two to wear, but now you're not sure about them. I speak to a lot of people who have tried hearing aids and then given up on them. I had this reaction too initially, and Adam Chell explains why that might be: 'Even with hearing aids, the sound still isn't the same as if you had normal hearing. This means it might not feel natural and it takes time to get used to it.' Amplifon audiologist Jane Noble agrees: 'It's important for your brain to adjust to all the new sounds it has forgotten, due to auditory deprivation, while your hearing deteriorated. Unlike new eye glasses, which may only take a few minutes to get used to, hearing aids have a longer "getting acquainted" period.'

Micaela Sharp adds: 'I lost my hearing aid and while I waited for a replacement I got quite used to not hearing in full. I rarely wear my glasses either, and I have just adapted to less hearing (and vision) over time.' While I love my hearing aid, I had a similar experience during the pandemic. For the first time I was on my own for prolonged periods of time. While this negatively affected my mental health, it did wonders for my listening fatigue. I was in an environment I could control (my home) and this meant I could control the level of noise I was exposed to. Only watching TV that had subtitles and not having to interact with and listen to others was an amazing break for my ears, and hugely reduced the strain of constantly trying to hear. I found that, as the pandemic went on, I wore my hearing aid less and less, as I just didn't need it the way I do in a loud hearing environment. There were no coffee machines to talk over, or colleagues to try to hear while lip-reading, or background noises of any kind, and I found a real peace and contentment in the new silence. As anyone who is deaf will know, it is rare to hear absolute silence. I have two types of tinnitus, so 'silence' isn't exactly right, but it was the closest to a relaxing 'lack of sound state' as I had ever been in. Now that I'm wearing my hearing aid again, it has taken my brain some time to get used to the new level of sound, and I remembered the importance of persistence. There's still nothing like coming home after a noisy day and taking off your hearing aid to bathe in a muted sound level, though – it's as comforting as taking off your bra at the end of a long day.

Jenni Ahtiainen, owner of jewellery brand Deafmetal and a hearing-aid user, understands the need for persistence with hearing aids: 'I wish that people would give time for their brain to adjust when starting to use hearing aids. I had terrible headaches for over a year when I started to use aids. Brains need to adjust to the sounds again.'

Adam Chell agrees. 'The brain can adjust and gets used to the new sound. It's like taking your ears to the gym. The more you wear them, the stronger your hearing brain gets, and the more benefit you get from the hearing aids.'

Audiologist and Little Auricles founder Rita Kairouz's top piece of advice for new hearing-aid users is: 'Be persistent! It takes a while for your body to become accustomed to hearing aids. It won't happen overnight. Make sure you wear your hearing aids consistently and you will get a lot more out of them.'

Comedian Angela Barnes recalls her hearing aids being sore to wear at first. I had a similar experience – the top of my ear and entrance to my ear would ache, as it wasn't used to having something there. And this persistence isn't just needed when you first get hearing aids; you will go through the same process of adjustment whenever you get new hearing aids.

Hearing aids and our appearance

Of course we are all well-rounded individuals who aren't overly obsessed with shallow things like our appearance. However, looking good makes you feel good, and anything that might change that can knock your confidence. Amplifon audiologist Jane Noble explains that many of her clients 'assume that hearing aids will be big and bulky, not knowing that nowadays most are quite small and discreet'.

Audiologist Adam Chell has some sage advice.

> If it's about self-image, try to flip it on its head. How would you feel if your friends got a hearing aid or if your partner got one? Would you care about how it looked on them? Would it affect your relationship with them, or how attractive they were? The chances are, you probably wouldn't care too much. But what you would care about is that they could engage with you better and join in more conversations with the hearing aids.

These are excellent pieces of advice. And listen, a hearing aid can't make you look any worse than that haircut you had in the 1980s, or the dress you thought made you look like a movie star when you were thirteen, but on reflection you looked like you had gone to a fancy dress party as an angry bull terrier. On top of that, neither the haircut nor the dress gave you any actual life benefits, like helping you communicate with hearing people, noticing when the doorbell goes, or helping you feel less isolated. Just saying.

Adam Chell goes on to say:

> Making hearing aids 'invisible' has been drummed into society by hearing-aid manufacturers and hearing care providers for decades. Although this is starting to change, a lot of the damage is done. When you suggest you need to hide something, it indicates that you should perhaps feel shame

or embarrassment. However, there is something magical happening at the moment. We are seeing a shift in perspective, and hearing aids are now matching expectations when it comes to self-image. Also, 'hearing aid' is an outdated term because they are so much more than that now. That's why I refer to them as hearing tech or hearables (like wearables).

So openly showing off your hearing aid – or hearable – could actually be fashionable now – hurrah!

So, if hearing aids are in and we want to show them off, how can we facilitate that? In the children's books I have written, which have deaf protagonists, the heroines always have colourful hearing aids. In fact, like children's glasses, children's hearing aids are way more exciting than adults' ones, with manufacturers creating bright colour options and personalisation. In my book *Harriet Versus the Galaxy*, Harriet's hearing aid is bright green, just like a bug, and in *The Night the Moon Went Out*, Aneira's hearing aids are red. I actually found myself becoming jealous of the characters I had created, as I could only find skin-coloured hearing aids, or silver and gold. (There was also a noticeable lack of diversity within what was called 'skin-coloured'.) I was very excited when Amplifon told me they could order me a bright pink Widex hearing aid! Finally I had something worthy of showing off. I was interviewed by the *Daily Express* and said, 'One day I want a Vivienne Westwood hearing aid, like you can get Burberry glasses.'[23]

Even though I'm still waiting for a call from the Vivienne Westwood team, I was excited to discover that hearing-aid jewellery is available. Jenni Ahtiainen, the founder of Finnish hearing-aid jewellery company Deafmetal, had similar thoughts to me about designer hearing aids. She says, 'Why is it that if you have bad eyesight, you can choose from whatever kind of eyeglasses suit your own style, but if you have bad hearing, you're stuck with these medical-looking machines for the rest of your life?' Unlike me, she didn't just name-check her favourite designer and wait for their call; she did something about it herself. 'First I made a small holder around the hearing aids (from leather), and then I hung some leather strips from the holder. And suddenly, the hearing aids felt more like mine. They looked like me. I looked like me.'

For Jenni, that moment was the beginning of a successful international hearing-aid jewellery business that helps hearing-aid users all over the world to customise their hearing aids and make them feel more like them. Similarly, Rita Kairouz, audiologist and founder of Little Auricles, an Australian hearing-aid jewellery brand, explains: 'People are excited about the prospect of not having to hide their devices any more, which is exactly what we are aiming for.'

I remember meeting Jenni Ahtiainen for the first time when I asked to interview her for this book. She was on a brief trip to the UK, and I managed to catch her for a couple of hours one night after a day of meetings. She walked into the restaurant with a Viking-style long plait, the sides of her head shaved, dressed all in black, with tattoos, and a huge smile on her face. Her hearing aids were adorned with her own jewellery designs: silver hanging chains ending in black leather which cupped her earlobes and secured to her ear piercings. She looked effortlessly and wonderfully cool, and her hearing aids were a cohesive part of that. After the interview portion of our meeting was over, we ended up chatting for hours. This is one of the best things that being deaf has brought me: I've met so many incredible people like Jenni. I wear her hearing-aid jewellery –

and not only do I look hella stylish doing it, but the jewellery connects to my ear piercings and helps to keep my hearing aids secure (they can ping off if I wear a mask, for example). I love them so much. In fact, Jenni and I are working on our own hearing-aid jewellery range! So there you go – being deaf has even helped me to become a jewellery designer!

Vivienne Westwood – the icon – died whilst I was writing this book. RIP Vivienne and thank you for your vision.

Chapter 6

What to expect at a hearing-aid fitting

I remember getting a phone call – yes, that's a phone call, despite me needing a hearing aid – to invite me to my NHS hearing-aid fitting. I had no idea what to expect. I was actually planning my wedding at the time (I'm now divorced. Don't worry, I'm fine), and I remember having more fittings for my wedding dress, which I wore for less than twenty-four hours, than for my hearing aid, which I wear every day. Luckily, at a hearing-aid fitting, unlike a wedding-dress fitting, you don't have to wear a matching nude set of bra and pants. I guess you can if you'd like, but it's not a requirement, and you definitely shouldn't show your audiologist your underwear.

This chapter is all about getting a hearing aid fitted. We already know that cochlear implants and BAHAs are implanted during an operation, so the same information won't apply there, although the new levels and types of sound will still be overwhelming and take some getting used to.

Audiologist Adam Chell explains:

> A hearing-aid fitting is the process of matching the technology to your unique hearing profile. Your hearing profile incorporates many things such as hearing ability, ear shape, cognition, dexterity and personal preferences. We can make a hearing aid as simple or as complex as you want. I'm not likely to set

up a hearing aid the same for a housebound ninety-four-year-old as I would for a thirty-six-year-old athlete, even if their hearing tests are the same.

When Adam told me this, I spent a good few minutes wondering if I'd be closer to the thirty-six-year-old athlete or the house-bound ninety-four-year-old. I settled on a fifty-fifty split.

Amplifon audiologist Jane Noble says:

> Hearing-aid fittings typically last an hour. During this time, the audiologist will adjust and set your hearing aids using real ear measurements, ensuring the aids are set to the correct level based on your hearing and ear canal side. They will also talk to you about management and care and how to effectively get used to wearing the hearing aids and changes you might have to overcome.

I would advise anyone going for a hearing-aid fitting to bring a notebook and pen: you will be given a lot of information, and I remembered less than 20 per cent of what I was told. Also, remember that the fitting is for *you*. Ask all the questions you need to (write down the answers), go over the cleaning/inserting process if you need to, and be honest about any concerns. I think I was still in shock from my initial test results, so I was just trying to get through my fitting without crying, rather than actually thinking about the fact that this hearing aid was my new best friend. You get more intimate with your hearing aid than a lot of partners: you see them every day and you rely on them in certain environments, so your introduction to one another is more important than you might first assume. But the main point of a hearing-aid fitting is to ensure that your hearing aids fit well and you know how to use them, including inserting them, cleaning them and maintaining them.

Another important thing to note for your fitting is that getting your hearing aids is overwhelming. Jaipreet Virdi remembers getting hers: 'I was fitted with my first analogue behind-the-ear hearing aids. They were large but, with them, my auditory world changed once again: I could discern between different sounds, hear my parents' voices clearly, and even understand television'.[24]

8 top tips for living with your new hearing aid

1. Book your appointment at a time when you can go straight home afterwards and do relaxing things for the rest of the day.
You are basically giving your brain a big workout when you get your new hearing aids, so you don't want to have to work or concentrate on anything too hard after you get them.

Comedian Angela Barnes remembers: 'It was a lot at first. Initially my audiologist set [my hearing aids] at 60 per cent, and then I had to go back and he turned them up.' Many audiologists will do the amplification in stages, and each stage can be overwhelming until your brain gets used to it.

2. Bring someone with you to the appointment, if you can.
They don't need to sit in the room with you when you get your hearing aid, but having someone around afterwards for support will be useful, as the new levels of sound can be very disorientating. You may need to take breaks on the

journey home, go somewhere quiet for a few moments, or even just tell someone what's going on for you, so having a friend with you can help you feel safer at this vulnerable time. I wouldn't advise going to a coffee shop or for lunch with your friend after your fitting, as these noisy environments will be almost unbearable: everything will seem incredibly loud until your brain gets used to the new, amplified level of sound. If you think about isolating during the pandemic it may help you to understand. Being at home in a noise-controlled environment for long periods of time, our brain and body got used to the new normal. Once we no longer had to isolate and could venture out into the world again, whether to a supermarket, on public transport or out for dinner, we were suddenly assaulted by all the sounds, smells, people and choices that we had forgotten about. Getting a new hearing aid is a lot like coming out of lockdown: it's exciting, but overwhelming, and the best thing to do is take things slowly.

3. Get lots of sleep.
Your brain will be going through a lot, so make sure you get the rest you need.

4. Have fun experimenting.
While loud sounds might be overwhelming, you will be excited by sounds that your hearing aid reminds you exist, or that you can hear more clearly. Asking a friend to stand outside and ring the doorbell while you test if you can hear it and from how far away is an interesting one. Going outside in the quiet morning and listening can be fun. Seeing how much lower you can turn the volume down on your

TV (with subtitles, of course), turning your back to a friend and asking them to speak and seeing how much you can understand without lip-reading cues, and trying a phone conversation with your hearing aid (if you have mild/moderate hearing loss) are all nice first-week testers.

5. Connect your hearing aid to your phone.

After a couple of days of enjoying ambient noise, it might be time to connect your hearing aid to your phone (if you have Bluetooth capability). If you have been struggling with the new experience, this should get you excited about your hearing aids again. Talking to a friend on the phone via your hearing aid, playing music/a podcast or even watching Instagram videos without a partner hearing them too will surely make you smile. The trick is to remember that your phone is connected to your hearing aid. Especially when you're trying to show someone a video of your dog saying 'I love you' and they are watching a silent video of a dog while looking at you strangely. Yes, this may have happened to me . . .

6. Don't expect too much of yourself.

While you will – hopefully – love your new hearing aids, you won't be on top form for at least the first week. Getting accustomed to the new level of sound takes time, so don't book your hearing-aid appointment a week before a work deadline, change of job, or big event you are organising. You will feel off-kilter – and that's okay. Take your time and don't push yourself too hard. The experience of getting hearing aids might be more emotional and overwhelming than you thought it would be.

And two further tips from audiologist Adam Chell (if, like me, you missed a lot of the useful information you were given at your fitting appointment):

7. Cleaning hearing aids

A great way to clean the end of a hearing aid is to get some kitchen roll and squirt a little bit of alcohol hand sanitiser (minimum 70 per cent) on it. Rub the sanitiser in and it creates an alcohol wipe. You can then rub the hearing aid and the end of the hearing aid with this wipe. It dries quickly and doesn't saturate the hearing aid with liquid.

I have tried this, and it works brilliantly. When you get your hearing aid, you are usually provided with a cloth and brush for cleaning it: however, I have found that the alcohol wipe option works much better for me to reduce infections.

8. Changing the batteries

If you use batteries in your hearing aids, sometimes the batteries get mixed up when you're changing them. Which is the old and which is the new? To find out, all you have to do is drop the hearing-aid batteries on a hard surface. The one that bounces most is the older one.

Thanks, Adam!

My hearing-aid fitting

My first hearing-aid fitting was through the NHS, although later I went private for hearing tests and new hearing aids. I remember arriving at a looming glass building near London Bridge Station. I felt apprehensive. I remember thinking I would get the hearing aid, but I could just not wear it if I didn't want to. I waited patiently, probably scrolling on my phone, in a carpeted waiting room until an audiologist stepped out of her room to call my name. Yes – again, my name was called, rather than appearing on a screen, even though I was waiting to be given a device to enhance my hearing. I mean, come on!

I wasn't sure what a fitting would entail. I hadn't even googled the procedure as at the time it still didn't feel real. Would they measure my ear? Was it anything like a wedding dress fitting? Should I wear high heels to see how the hearing aid looks when I'm two inches taller? No. It turns out that having a hearing aid fitted is remarkably like putting in a tampon for the first time. If you've never had the pleasure, don't worry. I'll explain.

I was given a RITE hearing aid in a nude (white person) colour. The section that goes behind the ear was about the size of a non-applicator tampon and peach-coloured, with a clear tube with a wire coming out of the smaller end, which led to a clear earbud. The audiologist showed me the device then plugged it into her computer to be calibrated with my previous hearing test. After this was done, she put the hearing aid in my ear, which was fine, if a little bit tight, and played some beeps and white noise through the hearing aid to check if I could hear them or if they sounded too loud.

The sound came gradually through the hearing aid as we worked through the tests, sounding a lot like speech coming out of a radio speaker. It was as if 'normal' sounds had been digitised; they didn't sound exactly the same as they did without my hearing aid. Everything did sound louder, but in the acoustically dampened room I didn't get the full impact of just how loud everything was right then. The next portion of the fitting involved the audiologist taking the hearing aid back out of my ear, showing me how it worked (how to turn it off and on, how to change the batteries). Then she asked me to put it back in my ear myself. This was the tricky bit. I had put earphones and even earbuds (for cleaning, which you shouldn't actually use) in my ear before, so I imagined this part of the fitting would be a walk in the park. How wrong I was. This is where we come to the tampon application metaphor, which is honestly the most similar experience I can come up with. In both scenarios, you know where the hole is and you understand from diagrams/advice where the device (hearing aid/tampon) is meant to go, but when you have to do it yourself, all those diagrams go out the window and it's suddenly a very confusing and fiddly business. I can't tell you how many times I tried to get the hearing aid into my ear, but I can tell you that it felt like I was trying for hours, and I was getting redder and redder. As a comedian and actor, I've done some silly things in my time. I would say I don't embarrass easily, but this had to be one of my most embarrassing moments. I was gob-smacked by the fact that I just couldn't get the earbud into my ear at the right angle for it to stay there without the back of the hearing aid falling forward. All the time, my audiologist just sat there silently staring at me. How could it be this com-plicated?! A couple of times she even put the hearing aid in for me, but that wasn't really helping. It turns out that advising me to put the earbud in first and then to loop the rest behind my ear was throwing me, as the hearing aid would not stay put! To this day I still put my hearing aid in the other way round, looping the back round my ear first then putting the earbud in place. Don't worry, it's not that hard – I do it now with ease, so it definitely had something to do with the high-pressure environment at that hearing-aid fitting. Plus, ear holes are a lot like vaginas: you can't represent them all on a diagram. It may look like a 45-degree angle on the instructions, but yours may be a different angle, and you just need to find your personal inclination.

The time I spent fingering my own ear while someone silently watched was not how I expected my hearing-aid fitting to end. It would have been better if, like the first tampon insertion, my mum had been waiting on the other side of the toilet door and shouting 'Did you do it? Is it in?' rather than an audiologist making eye contact with me as I fumbled. I rushed through the rest of the appointment, embarrassment still clinging to my ear and face, then hurried to the ladies' loos. No, not to change my tampon; just for a moment of solitude in a safe haven.

A safe haven? With my new hearing aid (I'd finally got it in, and I was keeping it in there now), my safe haven had become a nightclub of white noise and what sounded like white-water rapids. I retreated inside a cubicle and took a deep breath. I slid across the lock on my cubicle door, which set off a gong-like reverberating sound. Two women walked in, screaming at each other about what they wanted for lunch. Then the toilet started to take off, sounding like it was inside a rocket bound for space . . . Yes, you did read that right. Full disclosure? We didn't take off, but for a moment I genuinely feared for my safety and immediately took up a crouching position, holding on to the toilet bowl (which, incidentally, tells you exactly what sort of person I would be in an emergency). Turns out there wasn't a rocket nearby; one of the screaming women was using the hand dryer.

It might sound amusing now, but at the time, I was not amused. I felt confused, frustrated and utterly overwhelmed by this new environment. It felt like new walls of sound were hitting me, one after the other, and my head hurt. Of course, I reasoned, a toilet would be loud; I just needed to get outside. Outside would be better. Quieter.

Stepping on to the pavement, I flattened myself to the wall to avoid the car coming at me. However, it wasn't coming at me, it was driving slowly past on the road. I could hear every driver in London beeping their horns, only punctuated by motorbikes with racing-car engines. Music flared out of a car window so loud it was as if it was playing inside my head. Is this how everyone heard the world? I wondered. How could they cope with it? It was amazing, tiring and overwhelming all at once.

Of course, that level of sound is not how everyone experiences the world; it was my brain being flooded with new audio information. It turns out my hearing aid wasn't even turned all the way up, so once my brain was used to things and the sound had levelled out, I had to go back to have it turned up again. While I was thrilled to be able to hear more clearly, it was a very tiring experience that I just wasn't prepared for at the time.

For this book, however, I have interviewed people who had much calmer experiences. Some people's audiologists actually took them out on to the street with their new hearing aid and got them to walk up and down a few times so they had someone with them. When I went privately a year or so later, my audiologist brought me into the building's canteen so I could experience the level of sound with her, and she explained to me what was happening. I don't want to blame the NHS – they do brilliant and important work, and it's not a case of 'the NHS is no good for hearing aids', but I do think it is useful for audiologists and GPs to know what it's like as a person getting your hearing aid for the first time. It is a lot to deal with. Any support we can get at that time is so useful. I understand that private audiologists are paid more and have more time for each appointment. I would advise you to go private if you have the money, but it is so important that hearing aids are still available on the NHS for those who can't afford them. Everyone should have access to hearing aids if they need them.

So I get my hearing aids and off I go?

Yes and no. Amplifon audiologist Jane Noble explains: 'It's very important to go back for regular follow-ups and checks to ensure your hearing aids are performing well. Annual hearing tests and adjustments will ensure your hearing aid is always performing at its best for your hearing levels.' However, you do pretty much get your hearing aids and carry on with your life. To begin with, you only wear them for a few hours a day, as you build up to wearing them all day. The sound will level out and any soreness you have around your ears will calm down too – it's just like getting new shoes. The impact of getting a hearing aid really can change your life for the better.

Amy Morton remembers: 'When I was fitted with my hearing aid, I went from quite a reserved child to bright, engaging, and embracing the fun. The transformation was quite marked, and I accepted it fully, with no issues with taking [my hearing aids] out or putting them in. Much to my parents' relief, I accepted them instantly and off we went!'

Once I was over the initial shock, I soon started to love my hearing aid, especially when I got one that streamed music and could be controlled by my phone. It definitely gave me more confidence in social situations and alleviated some of my concentration fatigue too.

Part 2
Communicating

Chapter 7
Sign Language

BSL stands for British Sign Language. There is also American Sign Language (ASL) in the USA, Irish Sign Language in Ireland (ISL), Chinese Sign Language in China (CSL) and so on. Just like oral languages, each country has their own sign language, which includes signs influenced by culture, history and even local slang. These languages are incredibly important to the Deaf community, and should be preserved. The British Deaf Association (BDA) states that over 87,000 Deaf people in the UK use BSL as their preferred language:

> BSL has been in use for hundreds of years. The first printed account in the UK of its usage was recorded in John Bulwer's *Chirologia – The National Language of the Hand* in 1644. Before that, in 1595 Richard Carew first recorded an observation of sign language in use between two Deaf people.

So it's not a new thing by any means. I am learning BSL, and it takes years of study, practice and immersion to become fluent. The actor in me is drawn to the language because of its facial expressions and the creativity of signs. My BSL lessons are fun, like an acting class, and I already feel that I am more honest when I communicate in BSL, due to the physical aspects of the language. Currently I tend to use the sign language I know at the same time as speaking, which means I'm communicating using Sign-Supported English (SSE). When actor Rose Ayling-Ellis was on *Strictly Come Dancing* she often used SSE while speaking; however, at other times she uses BSL. SSE is different from BSL, which has its own sentence structure, and which differs from the structure of spoken English. Actor and BSL user David Bower explains this much more beautifully than I can:

> Sign language is a very poetic language, and is able to express qualities and ideas in unique ways that are distinct from the spoken languages. It follows a different path from inspiration or thought to articulation and expression, from thought to expression. It is a very sincere language. If there is already a language of the mind and a language of the heart, then maybe Sign is the language of the soul.

You can see an example of the structure of sign language written down in model and activist Nyle DiMarco's book *Deaf Utopia*. Nyle is American, so he signs in ASL and uses 'ASL gloss' in his book as a way to denote the more direct ASL translations. An example he uses is this sentence in ASL gloss: 'ME TRY-TRY FIGURE-OUT BRAIN TEASER TEN MINUTES.' The repetition of 'try' emphasises the effort, and the hyphen is used for two words in written English that have one sign. If sign language such as BSL or ASL is your first language, you can see why communication in written English takes some translation.

One of the first things you learn in BSL classes is how to sign your name and ask others their name. In spoken English I would ask 'What is your name?' but in BSL I would sign 'Your name what?' So, you see, BSL has its own structure.

It is important to note that I am not fluent in BSL, so much of this chapter has been informed by the Deaf people and BSL users I have interviewed.

IMPORTANT: Makaton is not the same as BSL or SSE. Deaf people do not use Makaton.

If I had a pound for every time I said I was deaf and also an ambassador of RNID and someone told me they can sign in Makaton, I'd be rich. Makaton is great, and it's great that people learn it, but it is *not* the same as BSL, so telling a deaf person you know Makaton is like telling an English person you know French. Yes, there are some similarities in the signs, just like oral languages have similar words, but they are different languages.

Here is a description from the Makaton website:

> Makaton is the UK's leading language programme for adults and children with learning or communication difficulties. It is also used by everyone who shares their lives, for example, parents and other family members, friends and carers, and education and health professionals.
>
> Makaton helps people living with:
>
> - Autism
> - Cleft lip and palate
> - Developmental language disorder
> - Down's syndrome
> - Global developmental delay
> - Multi-sensory impairment (deafblindness)
> - Verbal dyspraxia.[25]

To reiterate, Makaton is useful to so many people; it's just not the same as the sign language used by Deaf people. In this chapter I will use a capital 'D' for Deaf. This is generally preferred by British Sign Language users.

Why isn't there a universal sign language?

I am embarrassed to say I asked this question early on in my deaf journey. It is a question that many hearing people, and some people with hearing loss, ask. The response to this is, why isn't there a universal oral language? British charity Deaf Unity explains that people ask this question: 'due to a lack of understanding, a level of ignorance on the part of language learners, and an honest desire for a cohesive and thriving global Deaf community'.[26] I would agree. When I asked this question, I believed that life would be marvellous if we could all chat to each other, no matter where we came from, how deaf we were or what language we spoke, but in truth I knew none of the cultural nuances that come into play when that question is asked.

It might sound great to have one language by which we could all communicate, but when you look deeper into it, there is so much that would be lost. Language is developed over time, it is affected by cultural and societal changes and adapts to new technology and advances. These changes can vary wildly from country to country. For example, when Trump became president in America, new signs were created for him in ASL so that people could talk about him without fingerspelling his name each time. The leader of your home country has a different cultural reference to you than the leader of a country you don't live in, and each country's sign language adapts to take account of this. For example, one sign for former UK

Prime Minister Boris Johnson is a hand on top of the head, as if a toupee is flying in the wind! Sign language has its own slang and can differ from region to region in the UK, just like oral language. So language and identity are linked – and to lose one would significantly impact the other.

It goes even further, as sign language can also be affected by accessibility. Actor David Bower explains:

> Back in the late 1980s, sign language was still very grassroots and relatively pristine in its natural evolution as a language. Recent corporate business practice in sign-language access provision altered the evolutionary direction of sign language's organic growth so as to expedite the business model of sign-language access provision. I tend to stick to the original grassroots level of sign development.

So the teaching of sign language has also affected the growth of the language and the development of signs. As Rose Ayling-Ellis said in her Edinburgh TV Festival speech, 'You can always tell if someone has only just learned BSL or if they have grown up using it.' This is why most people recommend that you learn sign language from a Deaf teacher, who will have up-to-date knowledge of developments in the language. David goes on to say: 'I also pay close attention to International Sign Language, as I believe that that is where the world's Deaf culture is headed.'

While many Deaf people are resistant to a 'universal' language of signs (with the eradication of all other sign languages), there *is* International Sign (IS), which is something that has developed naturally through international communication within the sign language community. Charity Deaf Unity defines it as 'an invented system of signing to allow "cross-language communication" or "a translanguaging practice"', and says: 'There has been a call to stop the use of IS at international meetings as it erodes and undermines the core objective of many of these meetings: preserving the individual identity of marginalised people, which includes their culture and language.'

Deaf BSL teacher and SignSong performer Fletch@ explains: 'I feel that it [International Sign] tends to be used more by Deaf people who travel quite a lot.' Only time will tell whether IS will develop and become more widely used.

British Sign Language (BSL)

'BSL is important to ensure we can understand and communicate easily with everybody and remove the barrier,' signs Fletch@. Since I have begun to learn BSL, I have discovered how natural it feels. It really can overcome so many obstacles that hearing-focused environments create. Annie Harris, RNID advocacy officer, reveals:

> I love the ease of communication without any barriers. I don't have to strain and concentrate so hard on lip-reading. I can literally just switch off and still follow BSL. I don't have to adjust and be a 'hearing' person when I am communicating with my Deaf friends. It's when I feel most alive. Some signs are hilarious too! Boris Johnson comes to mind!

Deaf actor Nadia Nadarajah signs, 'BSL is another language – it's not English . . . It's not just "access" . . . When we get together socially we use BSL just like those that use spoken English. And, of course, the structure, grammar and syntax are different too.' Check out @signaturedeaf and @blackdeafuk on Twitter and Instagram to see examples of Deaf people signing in BSL.

In fact, in 2022 BSL became a legally recognised language in Great Britain, thanks to a campaign led by David Buxton of the British Deaf Association and supported by RNID. Annie Harris, advocacy officer for RNID, explains why this change in law was so important:

> We are getting tired of being treated like second-class citizens – we are constantly an afterthought. This recognition makes me feel that I am a person with rights. I deserve access to healthcare, I deserve access to public services, and to private services like the bank. With access I would be independent and have my autonomy without relying on someone to speak on my behalf. It may not all happen at once, but this recognition is an important first step towards equality and respect for deaf people, who can do everything but hear.

Illustrator Lucy Rogers says that BSL was her first language, before she started speaking. This is true for many young Deaf people, and sign language can be a fantastic tool to access communication. In fact, many people are campaigning for BSL to be taught in schools, whether or not pupils are Deaf. If I had learned sign language in school it would be so valuable to me now, especially after being told I had hearing loss later in life. As an adult, I have to pay to learn BSL, something that will massively help me communicate and bring me closer to the Deaf community, and which will be invaluable for my mental health. If you want to learn BSL as a Deaf person and believe it will aid your working environment (and of course it will, as it means you don't have to concentrate on listening the whole time), you can apply for an Access to Work grant (see p. 194 for more on this).

Amy Morton says:

> I am learning BSL currently and I encourage everyone to learn a little bit if they can. Depending on your hearing loss, it's not something you might need on a daily basis, but it's a great language in its own right and will give you another tool in your toolbox should you need it.

Rose Ayling-Ellis said it beautifully in her Edinburgh TV Festival speech: 'Hearing people can learn a new language – they can learn to sign. I can never learn to hear, yet I'm the one that's making 110 per cent effort to come to your world, to adapt.' I would advise everyone to watch Rose's speech from the festival in full – it's available on YouTube. It is incredibly honest, beautiful, and it will help hearing people understand the importance of accessibility and representation.

Lucy Rogers describes her communication journey as she grew up: 'I'm oral mostly now, but before I was seven years old I used to do more signing. However, I lived in a rural area with no other Deaf people nearby, so I learned speech therapy and learned to drop my signing to try and fit in with my hearing peers.' It's frustrating to hear that Lucy had to drop her first language to fit in with hearing people in her community. This happens all too often, instead of hearing peers learning sign language.

David Bower explains further: 'Children can often sign before they speak, because the vocal cords are still developing. It's fascinating to be able to communicate and know the thoughts of children at such an early age. Having a head start like this strengthens the child's overall communication and cognitive skills.' Sign language can be a fantastic first language for children from a young age, and learning hand movements means they are developing their motor skills straight away. However, there has been a lot of stigma and misinformation around teaching Deaf children sign language. Fletch@ reveals:

> All my life, none of my family would sign. They thought that I could talk and I could hear. My dad also told me that when they went to see a medical professional, they were advised not to sign as I would turn out mute. This was the reason they did not learn. Facing the communication barrier in general everyday life has a really big effect on my mental health.

American author, historian and Deaf rights activist Kathleen L. Brockway agrees: 'If parents choose to force a Deaf child to lip-read and keep up standards in the hearing world, that is exhausting for a Deaf child.' I know it's exhausting as an adult, so I can't imagine what it must be like if you are a child and all your energy is being taken up by growing, learning and driving your parents up the wall! She goes on to advise: 'If you learn early, the better you will become . . . It is our heritage language . . . I'm grateful my parents signed so I could communicate with them.'

BSL Interpreter Chelsea Fields describes her experience with her son: 'He used his first sign, for milk, at five months old, and by ten months old had a good vocabulary in BSL, which was very important when he became moderately deaf due to severe glue ear.'

It's not just young children who should learn BSL. Kathleen L. Brockway expands: 'I wish [hearing people] learned sign language on their own, without asking me to teach them.'

As we will explore, the burden for education is so often on the Deaf person, and this can bring its own pressures and repercussions for mental health. Some Deaf allies and interested parties do learn BSL on their own, and we'd love to see more people do this. People like Chelsea Fields take the initiative:

> I actually learned BSL as a hobby! I was eighteen years old and in full-time education, but browsing online I saw a video of sign language and was mesmerised by it. I started to learn some basics from home . . . Then I found an evening course for BSL level 1 in a local college. When I arrived for my first evening I met my tutor, a profoundly Deaf lady named Emma McAllister. Emma said I was a natural and took me under her wing. She whisked me off to the local Deaf club and I instantly fell in love with the Deaf world and BSL. I decided there and then I would go on to study BSL at every level possible and become a BSL interpreter.

Learning BSL

After Rose Ayling-Ellis appeared on *Strictly Come Dancing* (and won – sorry, spoiler!), Google searches for learning sign language increased by 488 per cent! It is amazing that so many people want to learn BSL, but it's very important that you learn from the right sources. 'If anyone wants to learn BSL, I always direct them to a Deaf tutor as I feel it is their language to teach, not mine,' explains Chelsea Fields. Activist Charlotte Hyde advises: 'You don't have to learn BSL to be part of the

Deaf community, but if a course run by a Deaf tutor is accessible and available to you then I would strongly consider enrolling.'

If you're interested in learning BSL, go to the Signature website (https://www.signature.org.uk/), as they have lists of accredited courses. There are lots of brilliant Deaf BSL tutors like Fletch@, who signs: 'I love teaching people sign language and watching them develop and achieve their qualifications. It makes me feel very proud.'

As someone who is currently learning BSL, I am surprised by how wonderful and intuitive it feels. Chelsea Fields tells me: 'I love that BSL is such an expressive language. I love that I can visually paint a picture with my hands. When I watch somebody sign a story, the whole story comes to life in front of me.' As a writer and storyteller, this side of BSL really appeals to me, and I was recently lucky enough to see Deaf performer Richard Carter do a signing story live. It was utterly mesmerising and I understood every bit of it, despite not being fluent in BSL. Similarly, Charlotte Hyde says: 'I understand that hearing people sometimes feel apprehensive about having a Deaf tutor, as they worry about communication. I think, however, they often don't realise that Deaf people have been communicating with hearing people their entire lives. It won't be an issue.' If you're still not sure about learning, Fletch@ wants to encourage you:

> It is very easy to learn BSL as it is such a visual language, and I feel it would be so useful and beneficial for schools to teach to students. I would encourage everybody to learn BSL and GO FOR IT! It can make such a difference in the Deaf community, and being able to communicate with somebody who is Deaf could really make their day.

Sign-Supported English (SSE)

Clare-Louise English from Hot Coals Productions tells me: 'Speaking and signing at the same time, using SSE, is my happy place. I wish the whole country could use SSE! I love this form of communication, it feels so right to me.'

SSE follows the structure of spoken English and includes signs for words like 'and', whereas 'and' is not used in BSL. Instead, you would just pause or continue with your list. For example, in SSE you would sign 'you and me', but in BSL you would just sign 'you, me'. While it is important to learn BSL, with its nuances, culture and grammar, SSE is a useful tool for communicating with hearing people, especially if, as a Deaf person, you learned to speak before you learned sign language.

Speaking to Deaf people who have interpreters

It's important to know that not all BSL users sign all the time: it is down to the individual to determine how they want to communicate. I find on the whole that, as long an interpreter is provided and the BSL user doesn't have to rely on family or friends to interpret, most people who are fluent in BSL would rather communicate using this language, but it's important to never expect this. Blogger Bethan Harvey explains: 'I never learned sign until I was in my early twenties. It depends what environment I'm in and who I'm with as to how I communicate. If I'm around my parents, I speak to them; if I'm around others that are Deaf or those that know BSL, quite often I will opt to sign.'

Deaf people who use BSL or SSE will often have an interpreter with them to translate any oral speech for them. Some hearing people have a mild panic when meeting a Deaf person with an interpreter for the first time, as it can seem confusing. I can understand this – I was confused about what the etiquette was initially. Should I talk to the interpreter or the Deaf person?

Interpreter Chelsea Fields advises:

> If you are ever with a Deaf person with their interpreter, always look at the Deaf person when you speak to them. It's natural for the hearing person to talk to the other hearing person, but this makes the Deaf person feel you're ignoring them. Look at the Deaf person – eye contact is important. Direct your questions to the Deaf person so they feel part of the conversation.

I sometimes find this difficult, as I like to play to my whole audience, but as long as the Deaf person is the main focus of your eye contact and communication you should be fine. To begin with, it may feel like you're being rude to the interpreter as you won't be looking at them the whole time they are speaking. Actor Nadia Nadarajah signs:

> I always advise: I've brought in the interpreter for *our* barriers. Why? Because the hearing person can't sign and I can't speak smoothly. So it means the interpreter breaks the barriers for *both* of us. I will always keep eye contact with the hearing person. Pretend the interpreter is invisible – they are there, but invisible too. I will always sign direct to the hearing person, but I do have to look away at times to make sure the interpreter understands, and then I'll turn back and maintain eye contact.

It is also important to speak. Just because someone is Deaf, you don't have to stand there in silence. If you've done this, don't worry, I did it too the first time I met a BSL user; I looked like a right melon.

When an interpreter works with a Deaf person, the interpreter will interpret, then voice over what the Deaf person is signing. Chelsea Fields explains:

> the interpreter will speak in first person as the Deaf person, so they will say 'I am really well, thank you, I've been busy with work this week' as opposed to 'He said he is really well, thank you, he's been busy with work this week.' The interpreter is the Deaf person's voice, so when you hear the interpreter responding, make sure you're making eye contact with the Deaf person still.

However, if you are a lip-reader like me, you may have to look at the interpreter while they are speaking, so you can lip-read what they are saying. I would, however, always turn back to the Deaf person to respond. It is, of course, important that both the Deaf person and the interpreter can see you and the interpreter can hear you, so they can translate what you are saying into BSL. However, the interpreter will usually be facing the Deaf person so they can see their signing. This means that spatial awareness when you're with a Deaf person and their interpreter is really important. As David Bower advises: 'It's not a good idea to stand with your back to a Deaf person in social situations. For the most part, we aren't really that interested in looking at your posterior, and when you do finally decide to turn around, you might be surprised to find that we have disappeared.'

You know who else you shouldn't turn your back on? Members of the Royal Family, so just treat us like the kings and queens we are and you will be fine!

But what if there is no interpreter? Here are some more tips.

- Relax. Remember that not all Deaf people rely on lip-reading, but they still want you to attempt to communicate.
- Don't shout. It doesn't help, as your voice gets distorted and less easy to understand. Plus, it's embarrassing.
- If you're struggling to communicate, type out what you want to say on your phone, or write on a piece of paper.
- But whatever you do, don't give up!

There's nothing worse than trying to communicate with a hearing person who just says, 'Oh, don't worry about it' and walks off. The Deaf person really wants to know what you're trying to tell them, so persevere! As Sarah Adedeji signs: 'Each individual is different. Just ask us and be patient. Do not dismiss us and refuse to try an alternative method of communicating; there is nothing more upsetting than being disregarded because we aren't initially understanding you.' Writing things down, showing videos to illustrate your point, using your own basic sign language and speaking clearly can all aid communication.

There is a lack of interpreters available for Deaf people and this can be a problem for Deaf people and their families. Lucy Rogers wants 'sign interpreters to be accessible everywhere for Deaf people who may need it in hospitals or other places. I don't want to see more CODAs [children of deaf adults] having to interpret for their dying parent in a hospital.' Access to healthcare is a huge issue for many BSL users, especially if medical environments don't book interpreters or use excuses like 'no one was available as it is so last minute'.

And it's not just healthcare; BSL users can also find it hard to access entertainment. Sally Reynolds (@info_sally on Twitter) recently shared her story on social media; she and two other deaf mums had booked tickets to a large concert for their daughters' birthday, then took the concert producers to court because they didn't provide an interpreter for the whole show, which is against the law. This lack of access is unfortunately all too common. Make sure you call out these injustices whenever you see them, and be an ally for BSL users.

If you'd like to book an interpreter, check out the NRCPD website (www.NRCPD.org.uk) to find your nearest registered, qualified interpreter.

BSL performances

Just like 'spoken word', when writers and poets read their words aloud to an audience, there is a thriving subculture of performers who use BSL. You can see some of these amazing performances on platforms such as Instagram and TikTok, which have made it easier for BSL performers to share their work more widely. BSL performers are different from hearing people who 'teach' sign language online (sign language should always be taught by an accredited teacher and/or someone with BSL as their first language).

BSL teacher and Deaf performer Fletch@'s introduction to performing came at nine years old. 'I didn't understand what music was or what it meant. My mum was playing a CD and told me that a lady was singing. She took out the booklet from the front of the CD case and showed me the words. She started the music again and told me to listen while she traced her finger along the words and I watched her lips. The song was Celine Dion's 'Think Twice'. As she sang along and pointed to the words, there was a part of the song where she sang 'baaaaaaby', and she showed me how the word was prolonged. For me, this is when SignSong was born, and this was the very first song I signed to.'

Many in the Deaf community are critical of hearing BSL performers, however, and prefer to support D/deaf performers. Fletch@ is a very popular Deaf performer – you may have seen videos of her signing at concerts on social media. 'I signed on stage at Wembley with Ronan Keating when I was sixteen and most recently I went on tour with Ed Sheeran.' Artists like Ed Sheeran have even shared videos of Fletch@ signing their songs at concerts to their fans. You might be wondering how a Deaf person can sign the music if they can't hear all the words live. Fletch@ works out her BSL translations and practises the songs before the show, and she has a hearing interpreter with her during the show to help her stay in time with the live music.

In 2022, I was lucky enough to host the National Signing Choir Competition – signing choirs from all over the country travelled to London to perform and compete. I had never seen a signing choir perform live, and it was incredible. If you haven't come across signing choirs before, the way they work is that music is played on a track (rather than sung, like with a singing choir) and the choir performs the words in BSL to the music. The choirs work together to sign in unison, inter-preting the words of the song into BSL. They are judged on their dance/choreography elements, performance skills and presence, as well as their props and costumes. Chelsea Fields, who was one of the competition judges, explains: 'Signing a song in BSL often means signing the words in a different order to how they are actually sung, so it can be difficult. But the end result is amazing.'

I thoroughly enjoyed the night, met some incredible people, and watched some awesome performances. I also introduced the Mayor of Chelsea and Westminster (who was handing out the trophies) as simply 'the mayor', as I forgot that people in office have names too. But I digress.

Chapter 8
Lip-reading

'Only 30–40 per cent of speech sounds can be lip-read, even under the best conditions', advises the National Deaf Children's Society (NDCS).

It is important to remember that not all deaf people lip-read. However, for most of the deaf community, including me, lip-reading is a useful tool to aid in oral communication.

But what is lip-reading?

Lip-reading teacher Lisa Cox explains:

> Lip-reading is a pretty bad name for it, actually! The Americans call it speechreading, which is more accurate. It means watching someone's lips, teeth, tongue, throat, cheeks, eyebrows and facial expressions to help understand what they are saying. Someone lip-reading also needs to use body language, context, anticipation, general knowledge, knowledge of language and rhythm of language to help. It is like a huge lateral-thinking puzzle where we need to use these clues to help our eyes to fill in the parts our ears miss.

Many people don't realise they rely on lip-reading until they discover their deafness or hearing loss. Journalist Liam O'Dell says he 'subconsciously' relies on lip-reading. Blogger Bethan Harvey agrees: 'I rely very heavily on lip-reading and reading body language. I do this instinctively without even knowing I'm doing it half the time. It helps me to have a better understanding of what is being said from watching someone's lip patterns and movements.' The more I think about it, the more I use lip-reading in everyday life – and even for social cues for when I can speak, for example. Lucy Rogers explains: 'Lip-reading is useful when I can't understand some people (they might have very low, deep voices or they don't really make much of an effort to pronounce their words well for a deaf person). Still, lip-reading is not perfect; I still miss out on a lot.' I find it difficult to hear higher-pitched voices, especially if there is background noise, and lip-reading can really help me in noisy environments.

Lisa Cox explains: 'I can understand 0 per cent of speech if I can't see someone's lips, but close to 100 per cent if I can see their lips and the environmental conditions are favourable (e.g. they speak clearly and the light is good).'

For the profoundly Deaf, lip-reading can be their way to get along in the hearing world.

Learning to lip-read

'Even if someone can understand just 5 per cent more of speech from lip-reading clues, that can be the difference between being able to join in and feeling isolated and wanting to go home,' says Lisa Cox. But is it possible to learn to lip-read? Lisa thinks so. 'Just about everyone has the ability to improve their lip-reading but, like any new skill, how much you improve depends on how much work you're willing to put in.'

Lip-reading classes have been on my list of things to do for a long time, but I just didn't know where to look. I was offered lip-reading classes via the NHS, but it was very early in my deaf journey and I was in denial that anything needed to change for me at the time. I also received a call about the classes, which wasn't the best way of communicating with a deaf person!

Today, lip-reading classes are available all over the UK. It is a good idea to make sure your lip-reading tutor is ATLA (Association of Teachers of Lipreading to Adults) qualified, and you can find your nearest class at https://atlalipreading.org. uk/directory-classes/

'Just watch people's lips as much as possible. The problem is that often we look away when we are hearing OK and only try to lip-read when we get stuck. Really, to improve our lip-reading skills we should be watching people's lips all the time – especially when we can hear. The brain is learning what sounds look like on the lips, so that in future, when the sound is not available, the brain can still remember what that lip shape sounds like,' advises Lisa Cox.

Lip-reading top tips

For lip-readers

It's important to have a good environment for successful lip-reading. The ATLA website has some top tips:

- You need to be able to see the speaker's face clearly to lip-read, so good lighting is a must. We can't lip-read in poor light or if a face is in shadow.
- Try to find a quiet place, away from distractions. Background noise is a real problem for us.
- Get the speaker to sit or stand at the same eye level as you.[27]

I find it useful to arrange the seating before I meet someone, with my need to lip-read in mind. If I'm in a group of people, I find it hard to be in the middle, with people on either side, as I need to turn my head to look at each new person talking, which means I may miss lip-reading the beginning of their sentence. Being in a TV panel-type environment can be difficult for this. I remember being asked if I had any accessibility needs when I was a guest on *Loose Women*, and not even considering the panel setup. Guests usually sit in the middle of the panel on the show, and it was only when we were live on TV, chatting, that I realised this was making it difficult for me to lip-read – especially under pressure. By the end my neck was definitely loose! By contrast, sitting on the panel for *This Week* with Andrew Neil, I hadn't been open about my deafness but the natural setup of the show – Andrew in the middle and two sofas on either side of him – meant that I could see everyone clearly (since no one else was on my sofa). I was sitting opposite Michael Portillo. Some people might not have been thrilled to see him clearly, but it was perfect for lip-reading purposes. I realise that not everyone appears on TV panel shows, but the same applies to boardroom seating or meeting-room seating at work, or even just sitting on a sofa in between your friends.

Victoria Sylvester, a teacher at Knightsfield School, a specialist school for deaf children, reveals, 'We have a horseshoe seating plan so that all students can see each other as they speak.'

Bethan Harvey says, 'Lip-reading isn't always easy, especially if the person talks very slowly, too quickly, shouts, turns away, or the lighting isn't correct. Sometimes even facial hair such as beards and moustaches can make it difficult.' While you can't reasonably ask someone to shave so you can talk to them – at least, not someone you don't know – a lot of accessibility will come down to you being transparent and speaking up for your needs. This can be hard to do, especially at the beginning, and you will find that you just put up with a lot of difficult situations and environments. Over time you will become more comfortable about sharing your needs, and hopefully those around you will become better at anticipating them too. Alternatively you may get angry and frustrated. While not exactly pleasant, this can be useful too, as it might push you to be bolder about sharing your accessibility needs. In a world where hearing people educated themselves on being deaf-aware and where workplaces had dedicated Access Officers this wouldn't be needed, but sadly, at the moment, this is not the case.

Lisa Cox explains, 'It can be very difficult concentrating on people's lips all the time, so you will need to build up the length of time you are able to do it for.' Concentration fatigue is common among the deaf community, and lip-reading is one of the contributing factors, so be kind to yourself and make sure you rest too.

For people who are being lip-read

'It takes two people to make a successful conversation, and the onus is on both of you to make sure that happens,' explains Lisa Cox.

Here are some top tips for lip-reading:

- Use everyday language – and get to the point (a good rule for life).
- Break up complex messages into shorter sentences.
- Pause more often – it gives us a chance to catch up.
- Keep the rhythm of the language flowing – but ask a fast speaker to slow down a bit.
- Speak clearly – and perhaps slightly louder. Please don't shout – it distorts your face, and can be painful for us.
- Be expressive – gestures, body language and facial expressions give extra clues to what's being said.[28]
- Try to avoid standing with the light behind you so your face is in darkness – this makes it impossible to lip-read you. Also, if it's late at night and the lighting is low, we won't be able to see your lips clearly.
- Be careful about letters such as 'p' and 'b', which are hard to lip-read. To help a lip-reader, you could use the sign for 'p' or 'b' when saying words that include this sound.

BSL interpreter Chelsea Fields explains:

So often, hearing people wander around while we speak. This is really difficult for a deaf person trying to follow your conversation. Speak at a normal speed! So often, hearing people panic and almost start to speak in slow motion, which is actually more difficult to understand because your lip pattern is different. Just speak at a normal pace. If the deaf person misses anything, they'll ask you to repeat what you said.

Lip-speaking

Lip-speakers can be used in similar environments to BSL interpreters, for deaf people who don't sign or who prefer to lip-read. Lip-speakers can be useful at small events such as a dinner party and at larger-scale events, such as lectures or award ceremonies. They will usually sit opposite the deaf person. Lipspeaker UK has a handy definition:

> A lip-speaker is a hearing person trained to repeat a speaker's message to lip-readers accurately, without using their voice. They produce clearly the shape of words, the flow, rhythm and phrasing of natural speech, and repeat the stress as used by the speaker. The lip-speaker also uses facial expression, natural gesture and fingerspelling (if requested) to aid the lip-reader's understanding. A lip-speaker may be asked to use their voice, thus enabling the lip-reader to benefit from any residual hearing.[29]

Chapter 9
Other technology

Technology can be an amazing tool, helping to make life in a hearing world that bit easier for people with hearing loss and deafness. If things like doorbells and alarms had originally been designed to be accessible, then we wouldn't have to purchase additional technology at our own cost, but there we are.

Luckily we don't have to hide our hearing aids in our hair any more (imagine all the back-combing) and there have been huge advances in technology (advances in hearing aids were discussed in Chapter 5) to make things accessible and exciting too. You can purchase accessories to enhance the performance of your heading aids, and these include TV streamers (these connect your hearing aid directly to the TV for clarity of sound), remote microphones, remote controls, telecoil systems and FM systems.

Connevans is one of the main suppliers of hearing tech in the UK, 'specialising in equipment for deaf and hard of hearing people and audio products' (www.connevans.co.uk). If you fancy a browse, you can go to their website.

Subtitles for TV programmes, films and videos

Subtitles or captions on TV programmes are not just useful for the deaf community; they're also useful for people who don't have English as a first language and people with other sensory conditions. I watch all TV and films with subtitles. You'd be surprised by how many shows have no subtitles available – or even, frustratingly, the wrong subtitles. Many people just won't watch TV without subtitles. Blogger Bethan Harvey explains:

> I always use captions and subtitles (they're permanently activated) whether I'm watching TV, my phone or another device. I find it so much easier to follow programmes, and I find it reduces my listening fatigue if I can read what is being said and what's happening so I don't constantly have to play catch-up or fill in the blank puzzles.

The deaf community and charities like RNID have spent years campaigning for comprehensive subtitles on TV. Annie Harris, RNID advocacy officer, says: 'Imagine the uproar if a programme didn't produce sound? Nothing happens for deaf people.' She goes on to explain that: 'It's extra-difficult when it's a popular programme and people are talking about it on Facebook, or in coffee-morning breaks with colleagues. You feel really left out. It's worse if you have watched a series . . . then the final episode comes on and it has no subtitles.' This actually happened recently on a popular reality-type competition show!

Comedian Angela Barnes recalls: 'My husband had never seen *Forrest Gump* so I bought that on BluRay. They'd subtitled the *Forrest Gump* voiceover that he does, but none of the dialogue.' So frustrating. It's as if TV channels are saying 'deaf people, this isn't for you' or 'we don't value you as consumers of our products'. It is important to note that when talking about subtitles on online videos on platforms such as YouTube, there are different meanings: open captions means that captions are the default, and it may be impossible to remove them. Closed captions for an online video can be turned on or off, and can even be customised.

Subtitles aren't accessible for all of the deaf community, though, as actor David Bower explains. 'I am an avid reader and enjoy using subtitles. But many Deaf people prefer just sign language.' While subtitles are incredibly important, so is BSL interpretation. Did you know that during the pandemic, the emergency announcements by the UK Prime Minster and government had no BSL interpretation?! This meant that the deaf community had to wait until the content of the speeches was reported in print media (which is not the first language of many deaf people) or until a charity like SignHealth had created content signing the information themselves.

I was proud to be part of RNID's recent 'Subtitle It!' campaign, which demanded that broadcasters make their content accessible and asked the government to make subtitles a requirement on more services. Mark Atkinson explains the charity's remit: 'Whether we're talking about barriers to getting hearing aids, or funding for new medical research, right through to how important it is to have high-quality subtitles so everyone can access popular TV shows, our voice is really needed at that national level.' The charity organised cinema screenings of subtitled movies over Christmas, and I welcomed audiences with an on-screen message about why subtitles in cinemas are so important. In fact, RNID advocacy officer Annie Harris says:

'Don't get me started on cinemas, where hearing audiences are *always* prioritised over deaf attendees. It's not right, and it needs to stop – 7 out of 10 times I turn up to see a showing with no subtitles, despite it being advertised to have subtitles.'

In 2022, I was part of the team that went to the Houses of Parliament to hand in the 'Subtitle It!' petition with RNID and RNIB (the Royal National Institute for Blind People). It was a scorching hot day – hello, climate change – and we met up in Westminster, donned branded T-shirts and held colourful 'Subtitle It!' signs aloft outside the Department for Digital, Culture, Media and Sport (which is a real mouthful as names go). Then we stood in front of Big Ben and the Houses of Parliament for a photoshoot to celebrate the moment. We were even told off by a police officer at one point, who thought we were holding some sort of incredibly small demonstration, and we had to convince him that our photo props were more along the lines of promotional posters than placards. We were all sweating heavily by the end, but luckily the photos turned out alright. I managed to get sunburn on my back because I had only applied sun cream to the front of my body, but at least I was doing something worthwhile, and it's all about suffering for our causes, isn't it? Annie Harris explains: 'The campaign is vital in gaining government's support, so that together we can make changes benefitting both Deaf and hearing-loss viewers.' All the legislation that the government needs to demand that channels input subtitles on their video-on-demand services is in place, but RNID is still fighting to get the government to actually do it! So far, this has taken over five years of work.

Theatres

Live captioning for live theatre

Stagetext is 'a deaf-led charity' that is 'passionate about making the arts a more welcoming and accessible place'. You can head to their website, https://www.stagetext.org/, to find accessible theatre shows and events in your local area. Since the charity was founded in 2002, it has been the leading provider of captions for theatres in the UK. For talks, their live captioners can 'deliver up to 300 words per minute at 99 per cent accuracy' – which is definitely nothing like the feedback I got after my touch-typing course when I was sixteen. From personal experience, I can tell you that their live captioners really can deliver. I have been a speaker at many live-captioned events, and it really enhances the experience. Yes, I would like people to watch my performance, but just like with subtitled films, captions don't detract from the performance; in fact, captions have even helped jokes to hit home if my delivery is a little off. Personally, I would much rather an audience feel comfortable and pick up on every word I say (whether audibly or via captions) than trying to piece together what they think they have heard from my talk or performance.

For events like theatre performances, Stagetext says, 'Open captioning is what we recommend, if we can make it work in the space, as it benefits everyone. We'll install purpose-built screens beside your stage for the whole audience to see. When selling access tickets, we recommend allocating seats with the best view of both the stage and the screen.'[30] Stagetext describes an alternative option, closed captioning on tablets or phones: 'Your venue may be better suited to displaying captions on personal handheld devices. The captions are created and cued in exactly the same way as our open captions. If your venue's seats can accommodate rests or stands to support tablets, this will improve the experience for caption users.'[31]

I went to an open captioned live musical performance of *The Rocky Picture Horror Show* recently and the captions actually added to the show. As you may know, *Rocky Horror* has some fun/filthy call-and-response moments that have built up over the years with its cult audience. I have only been to see the show live a handful of times, so while I knew a few of the call-outs, I wasn't aware of them all – but luckily for me, the theatre included the call-and-response moments in the captions! What joy! So the captions not only made the show accessible, they added to the fun.

Smart caption glasses at the National Theatre

You may have heard about the snazzy new technology being used by the National Theatre in London – 'smart caption glasses'. Stagetext explains: 'This solution harnesses emerging smart-glasses technology to display captions right in front of your audience's eyes. Smart-captioning glasses use automatic cues from the sound and lighting of a performance to time and display the captions. The captions themselves are prepared by an expert captioner in the same way as for a captioned performance.'[32]

I spoke to David Bellwood, Head of Accessibility at the National Theatre, about the glasses. He explained that the glasses work off 'the script, voice recognition and cue via the lighting and sound desks, so there is no provision for improvisation of dialogue'; the glasses will wait until the next scripted line.

He described the glasses as 'a solution that provides access to the widest number of performances', but added that the National Theatre still runs captioned performances with text appearing on a screen. I know some deaf people have found the idea of the glasses challenging, as it puts the burden on the deaf person who has to wear the glasses rather than making the whole environment accessible. The glasses also act as an identifier: if you are wearing caption glasses, it's a sign you have hearing loss or deafness, which makes some people feel uncomfortable. But if not glasses, what is the answer? I chatted to David about the future of accessible theatre, and he spoke passionately about 'embedding access from the beginning', adhering to the saying 'nothing about us, without us'. 'There has been an optimistic surge of deaf talent – actors, lighting designers and art designers,' says David, who believes that bringing deaf talent into the process from inception is one answer.

Personally, I would like to see a speech-to-text reporter hired for each show as part of the cast and crew recruitment process. He referenced the National's show, *Barriers*, which used creative captioning that appeared on the set. But what if you are not the National Theatre, and don't have money to spend on tech solutions? David's advice to smaller venues/theatre companies is to 'reach out to communities, ask for help, invite deaf people into your rehearsal room, and have fun with creative solutions to communication, even if it's a projector you get on eBay'.

Hearing loops

I must admit I have always been too scared – don't ask me why – to try a hearing loop, and no one really tells you how to do it, so here you go.

RNID explains on its website:

> If you use hearing aids, a hearing loop can help you pick up speech sounds more clearly, especially if you are further away. It focuses your hearing aid to pick up sound from the loop system microphone, rather than all noises in the area. This helps to cut out background noise.
>
> To use a hearing loop, you need to have your hearing aid switched to the hearing loop setting. Your audiologist may need to do this for you.
>
> Hearing loops are available:
>
> - In various public places. You'll know if there is a hearing loop if you see the 'T' sign displayed. You may need to check with staff that it is switched on.
> - With your landline phone.
> - With your mobile or smartphone.
> - For your home, if you want to use them with your TV or radio.[33]

To use the hearing loop on your mobile phone you will need to activate the telecoil setting. This is usually under Settings. On an iPhone, go to Settings > General > Accessibility.

Accessibility settings on mobile phones

Are you an Apple or an Android user? It's a big question. I've been both – sacrilege, I know. I was enjoying my Android life, but when it comes to connectivity with hearing aids, Apple is better, thanks to the iPhone's capabilities, plus accessibility. It's annoying, as we all know that iPhones are a lot more expensive, but almost all digital hearing aids will connect to an iPhone whereas many will not connect to Android phones. If your hearing aid won't connect to your phone there are assistive devices you can use, like a neck loop or ear hooks (available via the RNID website).

Accessibility settings are available on both Apple and Android products and offer useful skills such as a hearing health check, a warning if your music is playing too loud, vibrating functions so you don't need to listen out for noises, left and right sound balance for single-sided hearing loss, and increasing the treble, which can make it easier to understand speech.

Alexa/Google Home

While my mum thinks these devices are scary because they are listening in on our lives, Alexa or Google Home-type devices can be useful to the deaf community. If you struggle to hear alarms/doorbells, you can connect these devices to your Alexa or equivalent. Instead of you having to listen out for the high-pitched noise, Alexa can notify you by saying 'the doorbell is ringing' and sending a notification to your phone/TV to say the same thing. You do, of course, have to carry your phone around with you or be looking at the TV for the notification, but it makes it less likely that you will miss the doorbell ringing.

Alexa can go further by helping you communicate throughout the house without using sound. The Amazon Alexa website states: 'Alexa Subtitles let you see subtitles for Alexa's responses on supported Alexa-enabled devices with screens.'[34]

Keighley Miles from youth group FDC explains how this function works for her: 'My Alexa is fantastic and helps me a lot, especially with my children. I can make an announcement from the kitchen and an alert comes up on all our TVs that have Amazon Fire Sticks and lets my children know, especially my deaf son, that I'm calling them. They can reply and Alexa will show me what they are saying in subtitles.' You would have to make a decision to go, full Amazon, as a household, but this can be an incredibly useful aid for people in the deaf community who have a family.

Alexa has some more accessibility options too. The Amazon website says: 'Is Alexa talking too fast or too slowly? You can ask Alexa to adjust the speaking rate to your preference.'[35] You can also change audio playback settings to work with your hearing level: 'The Equaliser allows you to fine-tune the audio to suit your needs and personal preferences, as well as the room you're in. With the Equaliser, you can adjust for higher frequencies (treble), the mid-range frequencies associated with voices, and lower frequencies (bass) to get the most enjoyment out of your Echo device.'[36] You can also pair your Alexa device with another Bluetooth device, like your hearing aid (if it's Bluetooth-enabled), so that music and or notifications are played directly to your hearing aid. It's worth noting that, once it's been paired, your hearing aid may automatically connect whenever you're in range, so other people in your household may get annoyed that their music ends up playing through your hearing aid rather than the speaker! Google Home has some similar settings, plus you can silence 'talkback speech'.

Doorbells

Doorbells and alarms can be particularly difficult for deaf people, as we are relying on a sound to notify us of something. Don't worry, there are lots of options available to make life a bit easier.

You can buy Ring doorbells on Amazon and most tech sites: they range from £50 to £100 plus. The Ring doorbell does use sound to notify you that there's someone at the door, but it can also connect to your Alexa device to use Alexa as a backup notification system. Alexa can use sound to alert you or send a notification to your phone. I particularly struggle to hear the doorbell, and my dog Custard loves to bark at pigeons and even the moon, but not always when someone comes to the door, which isn't that useful! I use Ring and the Ring app on my phone, which sends me a notification and a video view of the person at the door. I can also talk via my phone to the person at the door, or activate a standard greeting if I don't want to come to the door, such as 'Please leave the package outside.' A video doorbell with a movement detector also gives me peace of mind from a security perspective, as I worry that I wouldn't hear an intruder coming into the house. I have a Ring doorbell for the front of the house and a Ring camera at the back of the house, which sends movement notifications to my phone. Mostly it sends me late-night videos of my cat smelling the plants, but at least they make me smile. Other doorbell cameras are available (I'm not paid by Ring to promote its products . . . although I am always up for making a quick buck, so if Ring is interested in sponsoring my late-night cat videos from my garden, I'm open to chatting!).

Alarms

There is only so long you can blame being late to work on being deaf until your boss starts googling 'alarms for deaf people' and you need to come up with a new excuse.

Blogger Bethan Harvey says: 'I rely on a few specialist pieces of hearing equipment to enable me to live an independent life. They are installed throughout my flat and include fire alarms, which are much louder than standard ones and link up with a vibrating pad that goes under my bed sheet. If the fire alarm is activated it will vibrate violently enough to wake me, as I would otherwise sleep through a fire alarm, which obviously would not be safe. I have a doorbell that is much, much louder than a typical doorbell: it connects to a specialist watch that I wear every day, which vibrates and displays a symbol of a door to notify me that the doorbell is going.' You can also buy specialist fire alarms that flash instead of making a sound.

For new mothers who may be worried about hearing their child cry, Bethan Harvey points out: 'I have a specialist baby monitor that sends a vibration to my watch, displaying a dummy symbol to let me know my little one is crying.'

Emergency services

999 BSL (www.999bsl.co.uk) is a new way to contact the emergency services if you use BSL, using a video relay service. It was launched in June 2022 after a huge campaign by

SignHealth. Its website describes the service as follows: '999 BSL is the name of the UK's first ever Emergency Video Relay Service in BSL. The service is available to download as a smartphone app (iOS and Android) and access as a web-based platform.'[37] This is a fantastic service. It means that contacting the emergency services no longer relies on being able to hear, because my hearing definitely gets worse when I am stressed – for example, in an emergency!

Remember that you can also text 999 to access the emergency services. You will need to pre-register with the emergency SMS service: see https://www.emergencysms.net/ for details. This is more accessible for deaf people (if you can text under pressure, that is).

Transcription services

If you like listening to podcasts, having a transcription available is really useful. My podcast The Divorce Social has downloadable transcripts, but you'd be surprised by how many podcasts – even those by large companies – do not.

Transcripts after a live event can also be really useful for people to read through anything they may have missed. This can be useful for work meetings, university lectures, presentations, wedding speeches – the list goes on. My maid of honour gave me a transcript of her wedding speech since, on the day, she was facing the other guests (the top table was behind the mic) so I couldn't lip-read.

There are lots of transcription services out there, so why not do some research to find the right one for you? The people I asked recommended Otter.ai (https://otter.ai/): 'Otter has your back – empowering you with real-time, accurate notes that are stored in one central, secure and searchable place so you and your team can be more engaged, collaborative and productive.'[38] Otter works via its website and the app. While it's not perfect, it is the most accurate transcription service I have found. You can try Otter for free, but if you're using it regularly you will need to upgrade your plan (starting at around £100 a year). It also integrates with Zoom, Microsoft Teams and Google Meet.

Software and apps

Video Relay Services (VRS) software can be invaluable for people who have BSL as a first language. Some government schemes have VRS built in, so it's possible to, for example, claim Universal Credit via the UK government website this way. Others provide the service for a fee by minute and invoice you at the end of the month. You can apply for VRS using an Access to Work grant.

Apps can also be a really useful way to support deaf people. Activist Charlotte Hyde says: 'I use an app called Cardzilla, which makes anything I type fill the screen. This allows me to order food and communicate without using my voice if I'm feeling tired or overwhelmed.' This is a great option to overcome communication barriers, as you can type a sentence or request then show the screen to the other person. Other people use notes apps to do the same, although the text is smaller with these.

Other apps, such as Otter, control hearing aids, and headline or video-editing apps to add captions to your videos, and decibel meters can also be useful.

Radio aids

A radio aid is a small microphone that usually hangs around the neck of the speaker. They are particularly useful in education environments. The Connevans website explains:

> In crowded situations or when a voice source is more than an arm's length away, hearing-aid users can find background noise levels as loud as the voice they want to hear. A radio aid system greatly improves the clarity of sound by allowing a human voice, or another desired sound source, to be fed electronically into the listening device, reducing background noise and sound loss between speaker and listener.[39]

They are often worn around the speaker's neck like a necklace – you just have to remember to take it off before you go to the loo! Activist Charlotte Hyde says: 'I also use a Roger Pen, which is an external mic that connects wirelessly through my hearing aids. I mainly use this in lecture and seminar situations.' They can cost over £1,000, but an education grant or an Access to Work grant should cover these. Children or young people can apply for a grant through the NDCS website.[40] Speak to your education provider to find out more.

The SoundPrint app

When I was writing this book I discovered SoundPrint, an app for your phone. I was amazed that it existed and was so excited to finally have something that would help me choose where to meet friends.

The founder of SoundPrint, Gregory Scott, explains what it is:

> SoundPrint is a crowdsourcing app for smartphones that enables users to measure the noise levels of whatever venue they're in (restaurant, bar, coffee shop, workplace, gym, church, etc.) and submit it to a publicly accessible database so others may find places based on how quiet or noisy they are. Users may also send in noise complaints or recommend certain venues to be added to SoundPrint's curated Quiet List of restaurants. SoundPrint then reaches out to the venues and offers them tips on how to optimise their acoustics or connect them with acoustic professionals.

Gregory has hearing loss himself and wanted to find a way to address noise pollution. I was delighted to find the app and I really relate to Gregory's story:

> I recall many times sitting at a restaurant table feeling completely lost in the conversation while others conversed and connected with each other. I would often nod my head in unison with the conversation, pretending to hear my companions when I could not, and then idly pass the time by entertaining myself with whatever fiction entered my head. At home, I would google 'quiet spots', which was often a fruitless endeavour. A place listed as quiet would often be blasting with music when I arrived with my date. This type of setting was not a great environment to talk in and get to know someone. As the struggle with dating was enhanced by not knowing where the quiet spots were, I started using a smartphone decibel meter to measure the venues, and would keep a list of quieter spots in my notes. Friends, those with normal hearing

and those with hearing loss, would continuously ask for these lists. This led me to create the app.

It is worth noting that the app started in the USA, so there is currently more data on there for US venues than UK ones, but I'm doing my best to add to them. The more people who download the app and do the 15-second sound checks at different venues, the more accurate data the app will have!

Live caption glasses: XRAI Glass

I was recently lucky enough to try one of the newest products to come on the market, XRAI Glass. Their marketing says:

> XRAI Glass is a pioneering software product with a mission to enrich conversation for hundreds of millions of people around the world who are deaf or have hearing loss. Users wearing phone-tethered augmented reality smart glasses will be able to read speech in real time through closed captioning. The XRAI Glass software converts audio into a subtitled version of conversation which will then appear on the user's glasses screen. The software's sophisticated voice recognition capabilities can identify who's speaking and will soon have the power to translate languages, voice tones, accents, and pitch.

The software is developed by XRAI and allows live speech to be tracked in real time with subtitles shown both on the phone and on the smart glasses, which are made by Nreal. The idea is that as smart glasses advance, the software can move with them. Since smart glasses have now been developed by Apple, Google and even Ray-Ban, it seems this is the biggest new technology trend. If we all end up wearing smart glasses, why wouldn't we want a pair that has live captioning capability? And this function could be particularly useful for the deaf community. Brand ambassador Jacqui Press explains:

> When trying on these glasses with XRAI software for the first time, it brought tears to my eyes because I was then able to speak to my father on the phone, which is something I've never been able to do. Once I saw how this gave me independence in being able to make telephone calls without relying on any support, especially as a mother making calls for my children to the school/doctor/friends, etc., it gave me the ability to be able to be included and connect with others as myself and not via someone speaking for me.

XRAI recognises the need for BSL interpreters and accessible events, but describes the product as 'a different way to allow access'. The glasses can be used for situations in which lip-reading would be impossible, such as phone conversations (the microphone picks up the phone audio), cinema visits and conversations in the dark, such as a late-night taxi ride with a friend. You can also buy the glasses with your own eye prescription, and they come with adaptable arms so they don't push on your hearing aids. XRAI ambassador Jacqui Press is deaf herself and understands that the onus is so often on deaf people to make the world accessible, rather than the other way around, but the fact is that interpreters often cannot be found at the last minute and these glasses offer an alternative. 'We are not helping deaf people; we don't need help. We are just making life accessible for anyone who needs it,' Jacqui explains.

These glasses and software are not just useful for deaf people; anyone who uses subtitles on TV could benefit from them. I believe these would work best in an environment where lots of people were using smart glasses so the devices wouldn't mark you out as a deaf person or 'other'. They are pricey, at £399.99 for the glasses alone at current prices, plus a monthly subscription for the software – but presumably if you were using them for access you could apply for an Access to Work grant to cover the cost, or your workplace could provide them. The glasses are still in development. I provided my feedback on my experience wearing them, and I'm excited to see where these could go. Contact lenses with live captioning could be interesting!

Part 3
Living your life

Chapter 10

Tinnitus

What is tinnitus?

Nic Wray from Tinnitus UK explains:

> Tinnitus is a sound you hear inside your head or ears, but
> there's no matching outside sound. It's often called 'ringing in
> the ears', but people can hear a wide variety of sounds,
> including buzzing, whooshing, humming or even snatches of a
> familiar tune or song. Tinnitus can be constant or it can come
> and go. People can sense it in one ear or both, or it can feel
> like it's coming from somewhere in their head.

Historically tinnitus was called 'singing in the ears', which I
prefer. My ear singer is, however, very bad at singing. If there
was an *X-Factor*-type show for tinnitus, my tinnitus would
definitely be one of those awkward audition videos that gets
shared on the internet. I have two types of tinnitus: a high-
pitched beep (let's call him Tinnitus 1), which is constant, and
a whooshing/scrambling noise brought on by loud noises (let's
call him Spider Tinnitus – all will become clear soon). I used
to make a joke about my double tinnitus: 'I have two types of
tinnitus because it was buy one, get one free – and I love a
bargain.' I said that on Sky News and got trolled heavily by
other tinnitus sufferers, who believed I was making fun of
them. But I wasn't making fun of them; I was trying to make

sense of my own experience and start a conversation about tinnitus in an accessible way, through humour. I am still surprised by how many people don't know what tinnitus is or who can't say the word (it's pronounced tin-it-tuss). Nic Wray from Tinnitus UK told me: 'Currently, the best estimate we have is that 7.1 million adults in the UK have tinnitus (around 13.1 per cent of the adult population). This doesn't include children – and we know that around 1 in 30 young people have clinically significant tinnitus.'

This isn't exactly a small number, so why don't we talk about tinnitus? It doesn't have the ageing connotations that deafness can have, so are we just scared of telling people that we can hear things in our head? The way mental health has been treated in the past, it's no wonder we're scared of opening up about something that no one else can see. I had only heard of tinnitus as a 'musician's condition' previously, so perhaps we don't like talking about it because we feel to blame for our tinnitus by exposing our ears to loud music/sounds.

In fact, tinnitus isn't a modern thing. You may know that Beethoven was deaf, but did you know he also had tinnitus? In a letter to Franz Gerhard Wegler on 28 June 1801, Ludwig van Beethoven wrote: 'My ears whistle and buzz continually, day and night.'

According to Wikipedia, other notable people with tinnitus include moi, Vincent van Gogh, Phil Collins, Eric Clapton, Will.i.am, Keanu Reeves, Barbra Streisand, Richard Atten-borough, Charles Darwin, Demi Lovato and Bryan Adams, who presumably got his in the Summer of 69 (sorry, I couldn't help it). So we are in a pretty fun group of people with singing ears, and I can't wait for us to meet up.

The first signs of tinnitus

Tinnitus is arguably easier to detect than gradual hearing loss: the first sign of tinnitus is the tinnitus itself. It's important to note that tinnitus isn't always a sign of being deaf, but it is worth having a hearing test to be sure. My deafness and tinnitus go hand in hand, which is cute, but many people will have tinnitus without deafness and vice versa.

Nic Wray explains:

> While we don't know for certain what causes tinnitus, these are some of the most common triggers:
>
> - hearing loss
> - exposure to loud noise
> - stress and anxiety
> - ear infections
> - ear wax build-up[41]

Please see your GP at the first signs of tinnitus, as things like ear infections and wax build-up can be easily treated and may even end your bout of tinnitus. Other types of tinnitus are constant and last throughout your life or come and go.

There were a few reasons I eventually went to see the doctor about my hearing, but one of the main ones was my tinnitus. I had heard of tinnitus, but thought it was something that people got after going to a loud concert, and that it disappeared after a few days. How wrong I was.

I had no idea that some people have constant tinnitus. Pop star Will.i.am said in an interview: 'I don't know what silence sounds like any more',[42] a description that feels very profound to me. Not knowing what silence sounds like is how I imagine new parents feel, but at least you can escape your children. However, when I take out my hearing aid I never experience complete silence, as my tinnitus is always with me. Having a noise in your head that no one else can hear is kind of terrifying, initially. You wonder if you are imagining it, you press your finger firmly into your ear and pull on your earlobe in the hope of shaking out this new sound. When it doesn't disappear, you simply try to ignore it. It feels like a stereotypical British reaction, doesn't it? 'Oh dear, there is a noise only I can hear and it doesn't seem to be going away. What should I do? Oh, I'll ignore it. It will probably be fine. Shall we have a cup of tea?' Four buckets of tea later, my tinnitus hadn't gone, but at this point I didn't even realise it was tinnitus.

You see, I thought tinnitus only meant a ringing in the ears – not like a phone ringing but like a high-pitched ringing. As activist Charlotte Hyde explains: 'My tinnitus sounds like the ringing sound effect they use when people have been in car crashes on the telly.' Charlotte has the classic TV tinnitus, but neither of mine sound like that so I thought it couldn't be the same thing. The word 'tinnitus' comes from the Latin for 'ringing', so I wasn't far wrong in my assumption. The Tinnitus UK website explains that tinnitus 'is not a disease or illness; it is a symptom generated within the auditory system',[43] but we don't know why so many different sounds are heard as part of tinnitus.

Tinnitus is a lot like how I imagine aliens will arrive – in that they will come in many different forms and upset people. Tinnitus UK explains that: 'The noise may be in one or both ears, or in the head, or it may be difficult to pinpoint its exact location. The noise may be low-, medium- or high-pitched.

There may be a single noise or two or more components. The noise may be continuous or it may come and go.' Basically, if tinnitus was a character in a movie, she'd be the elusive woman who saunters over to a group of people to say, 'I'll be whatever you want me to be, darling.' Then she'd kick their asses because they're bad guys and this is a feminist movie. My 'Spider Tinnitus' is not a ringing noise; it is more like a wavering, like the sound you get when you attempt to fan someone with a large book and you go in too strong, producing an audible whoosh of air. Mine is not constant but is brought on by loud music and loud environments like trains, which makes commuting even more fun.

So, since I thought tinnitus was just a ringing noise and all I could hear was a weird wavering and at this point I didn't think I had any hearing problems, I obviously assumed that I had spiders living in my ear – hence my nickname for it. It was the only logical choice, right?! Right?! I genuinely considered that a family of spiders living in my ear could be the cause of this new sound. I think I've spent too much time watching clickbait 'you'll never believe what was living inside her' videos on Facebook. You may be thinking that I'm exaggerating this for comedy effect, that I can't really have thought there might be something living in my ear, but I promise you I did. It was the only reason I could think of for this strange noise. If it wasn't spiders, I thought it must be some strange fly larvae – and writing that just made me shudder. In my defence, audiologist Adam Chell told me some of the strangest things he's removed from people's ears include 'cotton wool bud tips, popcorn kernels, toys and a moth'. Yes, those fluttery, ugly butterflies that are obsessed with lights – imagine having one of those in your ear canal!

I've never liked things going near or in my ear. I didn't even like my ex-husband kissing my neck near my ear – another reason for our divorce. I should make it clear here that this is not a sign of hearing loss. My dislike of things in my ear has nothing to do with my hearing and everything to do with *Star Trek*.

From about the age of twelve, I would always try to stay up as late as possible to watch naughty, post-watershed TV because it made me feel super-cool and grown-up. My mother was one never to cross when it came to bedtime, but my dad always tried to be the 'cool dad' (which was embarrassing when he was drunk and trying to tell me how great sex was, but incredibly useful when it came to bedtime). He would let me stay up late and watch TV with him. Mostly we watched sci-fi or the *Die Hard* movies, which seemed to be on TV constantly in the 1990s. *Die Hard* gave me a love of Alan Rickman, and the sci-fi made me hate anything going near my ear. *Star Trek* was our favourite to binge-watch late at night – this was way before Netflix and box sets and even before DVDs! We watched most of the *Star Trek* series, but they were never aired in the right order, which meant we had to do a bit of creative thinking to work out what must have happened in the previous episode. We weren't fans of the later series, which were better at special effects and make-up; the female captain was the best thing about those episodes. We liked the old-school Captain Kirk, Spock and the 'rife sexism' series of *Star Trek*. It was during one of Kirk and Spock's escapades in an episode with frighteningly little female representation that Russian crew member Chekhov was captured and tortured – using his ear. I vividly remember this episode almost twenty years later. Pavel Chekov was being held prisoner on an alien planet in a huge cave (most things happened in huge caves on alien planets, presumably as that was easier than creating new planet landscapes every episode). Anyway, Chekov's captor was trying to make him talk, and he did this by putting a fat worm-type animal – like the grubs they eat on *I'm A Celebrity, Get Me Out of Here* – in Chekhov's ear. Yep, he put an animal in his ear. It started burrowing in and wrapping itself around his brain, which was obviously very painful, and there was blood. Years later I read *The Hitchhiker's Guide to the Galaxy* and found out about the Babel fish, which you could put in your ear to understand any alien dialect – sounds mighty useful, especially for someone with hearing loss, as accents can make things difficult! Unfortunately my idea of animals in your ear had been ruined at age twelve by this *Star Trek* episode. That may be why I can't watch horror films to this day!

I did try to watch one horror film when I was fifteen. The film was *Halloween H20* and I watched it with my friends Holly and Nozomi with all the lights off – and something bad happened. Well, it was bad for me. Holly's house was on a very green and quiet estate and felt like a remote cabin in the woods, perfect for horror. We were also home alone because Holly's parents were cool and trusted us to not to do anything daft.

The film was so scary that at one point Nozomi took an ornamental bedpan off Holly's wall (yep, it was hanging on the wall – it was an historic kind of property) so we could defend ourselves. At one particularly tense moment in the film, when a murder was about to happen, Holly's dad came home very quietly and decided to surprise us by running into the room and shouting 'Boo!' As you can imagine, we screamed very loudly and, in the ensuing commotion, Holly managed to scratch my forehead. No, 'scratch' isn't dramatic enough.

Holly's thumbnail managed to peel a rivet into my forehead from eyebrow to hairline. This 'scratch' scabbed over and remained for weeks. It was there for our school trip to Shropshire, so in all the photos I have a sort of lazy Harry Potter scab. So please never invite me to watch a scary movie.

I still love sci-fi, though, even after that *Star Trek* episode, but I hate having anything in or near my ear. In addition, from then until the present day I sleep with my duvet pulled up over my ear in case something were to crawl in there while I was asleep and start eating my brain. I genuinely still do this.

Is there a cure for tinnitus?

No.

Sorry, I didn't want to give you false hope. Nic Wray explains: 'There currently isn't a cure for tinnitus, and it is the one thing that everyone living with tinnitus dreams about! Progress is definitely being made towards that goal, but it's hampered by a lack of funding, although it's not quite as simple as that – but more investment would definitely help.'

How can you manage tinnitus?

Finding out there is no cure for tinnitus might leave you feeling a mixture of dread and despair (I've been there), but there are things you can do to manage your tinnitus that can really help.[44]

- Stress management – like with most things, stress can make your tinnitus worse.
- Background noise while you sleep, or at quiet times, to drown out the sound.
- Caffeine can make tinnitus worse, so avoid too much tea or coffee.
- Mental health support from a trained therapist.
- Finding your community and sharing your experiences.
- Have a hearing test – a hearing aid could help by limiting the amount of sound going into your ear.

Don't buy pills to cure tinnitus off the internet, because they don't work. Nic Wray explains: 'There isn't a drug or supplement that you can take for tinnitus, so people shouldn't waste their time or money buying pills.'

My hearing aid really helps with my tinnitus, and this is quite common. Hearing aids can control the level of sound that is allowed into the ear, so this can help with tinnitus brought on by loud noises, like my spider noise. I rarely experience the spider noise tinnitus if I'm wearing my hearing aid, which is another reason I love her (yes, my hearing aid is a her).

Importantly, tinnitus can have a huge impact on your mental wellbeing. Some people with tinnitus feel like they can carry on with everyday life and not let it affect them too much, but it can be very distressing for other people, with a huge effect on their quality of life. Tinnitus can affect 'sleep, the ability to concentrate, and mental health – anxiety, depression and low mood often accompany tinnitus. Some people find it restricts their working and social lives and affects their relationships with family and friends,' explains Nic Wray. She goes on to say: 'Living with tinnitus can be relentless. Prior to Tinnitus Week 2022, we surveyed people living with tinnitus, and 87 per cent thought about tinnitus every day. One in ten respondents has had suicidal thoughts or thoughts of harming themselves since being diagnosed.'

That's why it's so important that we take tinnitus seriously. It is very important to seek help if you have tinnitus. You can see your GP and be referred to a counselling service, or seek private therapy to help. And there are also lots of support groups that meet online and in person across the UK. The team at Tinnitus UK offer free support and resources to anyone living with tinnitus – contact them on 0800 018 0527 or visit https://www.tinnitus.org.uk/. You can also find a list of local support groups on their website: https://www.tinnitus.org.uk/find-a-support-group.

In case you were still worried, there were no spiders or creatures of any kind living in my ears. Also, the worm creature I saw in *Star Trek* is fictional and does not exist! Phew!

Chapter 11
Living with hearing loss

People with hearing loss and deafness are, of course, human beings first, so the important thing to remember is the *living* bit. We live wonderful, full, interesting, successful lives – and you will too if you're new to the club. Yes, I've decided it's a club: there are no membership cards, but feel free to use my face as the logo (not that I am *the* deaf role model, but I could totally be a mascot, like the ones they have for the Olympics).

If you are deaf, though, some things make life a bit more difficult to navigate, and that's down to our society, which has been built without a thought for accessibility. If everything had been created to be accessible in the first place, then life would be much easier for the deaf community. When we are at home in an environment with subtitles, flashing/vibrating fire alarms, family members who know to communicate clearly/use BSL, and technology that aids us, our lives are much easier. We don't 'suffer' because we are deaf; we 'suffer' because an office environment/restaurant/university/transport service might not cater for deaf people.

Initially, I was very worried about what being deaf might mean and how it might negatively affect my life, but it's one of the best things that's happened to me. I love being deaf. I love my hearing aid – both wearing it and not wearing it, and enjoying the lack of sound (not silence, for me) I experience. It's only when an obstacle is put in my path and I have to jump over it or find a way to squeeze through it that I am reminded that the world isn't always welcoming to deaf people like me. As Keighley Miles from Families of Deaf Children says:

> Day to day you forget, because life is what it is, but then little things remind you, like when you're out with friends and they are on their phone talking and you think 'I wish I could just pick up the phone and talk' or when there's a programme you're really looking forward to and it doesn't have subtitles. It's all the little things people take for granted that I have never been able to do, and they don't even realise they have the luxury of doing them.

These reminders can be frustrating and draining, but remember that you're not alone. We are all in this together, and if we all strive together for a more accessible world then change will happen more quickly.

Hearing loss in childhood

Being an adult with hearing loss and deafness can feel frustrating at the best of times, because of the lack of accessibility, but if a child is going through the same things, it can affect their development. In the past, as has been mentioned, many families of deaf children were advised not to learn sign language to communicate with their child. Studies now show that BSL can be an excellent access point into all languages, including spoken English, and giving your child access to both languages furthers their development. For example, 'If children are unsure of a sign, they can always fingerspell the word in the air . . . This improves their spelling, as they have to use the letters of the alphabet to express what they are trying to say.' Learning BSL can also:

> broaden your child's vocabulary and helps them remember words as there is muscle memory involved. The more senses involved in their learning, the greater a child's memory retention will be. Furthermore, by seeing words in actions, it provides an additional way for children to recognise different words and phrases. At a young age, children are visual learners, so being able to see words in motion is a great way for them to retain information.[45]

Many parents also have to decide whether or not their child should have cochlear implants under general anaesthetic – or let their deaf child make the decision for themselves in later life. These choices can be hugely impactful to parents as well as being very personal, so there is no right answer here.

As a deaf child, navigating the education system can be trying. Blogger Bethan Harvey says:

> My mum clearly remembers my first sports day when I was in infants [school]. I took part in a running race, the aim being to run from one cone to the other, around the cone and back, but I didn't hear the instructions. Instead of running to the second cone and turning round, I got to the second cone and kept running up the school field. Teachers and my mum began shouting and calling me, but I couldn't hear them and kept running. My teacher who had taught me in reception was very aware of my deafness and came running up the field after me and explained, turning me back around (annoyingly, I had

been in the lead but because of continuing to run I came last. I still think I should've won that race).

Bethan totally won, in my opinion! The race should have been rerun, at least. If the first teacher had made sure her instructions were accessible, she could have ensured that Bethan understood the rules. This could have been done by printing out the rules and giving a copy to each pupil (not just giving a printout to Bethan, as this would single her out as being 'different' to the other children). Can you remember one mistake you made at school? How embarrassed did you feel? Well, think how Bethan felt after running the wrong way.

I remember learning debating at school. I got too involved in the argument and shouted, 'I don't know! I'm not the prime minister, am I?'

I shouted this at the most popular boy in my class, and all the other students looked at me as if I had slapped him. I went bright red and felt so embarrassed. That wasn't to do with my deafness, it was my heightened emotions (thank God I went into acting to channel all that!), but that embarrassment stayed with me throughout my time at school. If I could help another child avoid that level of embarrassment by making sure they understood my communications, I would always strive to do that – wouldn't you?

Accessibility doesn't just affect your social standing; it can also affect your actual education. Bethan Harvey says:

> I vividly recall struggling at junior and secondary school to keep up with my peers, missing information given by the class teachers, whether it was classwork and instructions on what

to do, or homework being given out. I would ask for repetition and/or clarification numerous times. My classmates would laugh and take the mick out of me, so I stopped asking. This resulted in me falling behind.

All children deserve access to education. To find out that in the UK children are essentially being denied an education because of easily rectifiable communication barriers is heart-breaking. Having a deaf parent can also affect a child's education: for example, if the school does not make events accessible, by providing interpreters at parent–teacher meetings and school plays. Keighley Miles explains:

I feel I haven't been able to be involved in [my children's] school lives as much as other mums, especially my oldest son, Oliver, who is hearing. At his school assemblies I can't hear anything, so although I try and go to them all, I don't actually know what is happening. Plus I can't pick out the single sounds of phonics so I can't correct him when he's reading, but luckily my [hearing] husband has been able to step in.

There are schools for deaf children around the UK, mainly funded by local authorities (so you don't have to pay for your child to attend), and you can look up their Ofsted reports just like you can for mainstream schools. Victoria Sylvester, a teacher at Knightsfield School, a specialist school for deaf children, says:

Based on our data, most pupils perform at or above their expected outcomes, which they would struggle to achieve in larger class sizes, with background noise and without additional support. Teachers use transmitters that connect to each student's listening equipment. We have regular interventions such as speech and language to support our students' development. We have maths and English tutors on site to hold one-to-one sessions with pupils. We have specific lessons every day to focus on different areas of need, such as mental health and deaf awareness too.

I think it's important to note here that many people I interviewed for this book believe that young deaf children should learn and use sign language: however, Victoria explains: 'We are an auditory-oral school . . . we complete daily hearing checks and maintenance of listening equipment, supporting our students with this and increasing their independence to take responsibility with their equipment.'

Many people I interviewed talked about the problems involved in advocating for your deaf child (whether the parent is deaf or hearing) and the educational politics sometimes involved in this. Bethan Harvey says:

I have many resources for my daughter, both for now and as she grows, to help normalise deafness and help her to be deaf aware, such as a whole variety of books and stories and a dolly that has a hearing aid and cochlear implants (this is currently her favourite toy – she carries her deaf dolly everywhere).

Deaf representation is so important for all of us, especially children. It's essential that there are books available showing deaf characters, and deaf dolls, such as the new deaf Barbie. This helps to make children feel that they belong and they're a valid and accepted part of our world.

If you feel you need support with navigating the world on behalf of your deaf child then the National Deaf Children's Society (NDCS) is a great place to start. It describes itself as 'the leading charity for deaf children. We're here for every deaf child who needs us – no matter what their level or type of deafness or how they communicate'. Their website, www.ndcs.org.uk, contains resources for parents, young people and teachers alike.

The impact of hearing loss

Hearing loss and deafness can hugely impact your mental health, as we will explore in Chapter 16. Having hearing loss can also impact your everyday life, by making it harder for you to access certain services. Mark Atkinson explains: 'Access to healthcare to manage hearing loss and tinnitus is something many people are really struggling with, and for profoundly deaf people access to all kinds of healthcare is often extremely difficult.'

Many GPs only allow you to book appointments over the phone, many have audio-based alert systems (like a GP calling your name in the waiting room, rather than your name appearing on a screen at the same time), and interpreters are regularly not provided at GP services and hospitals, so it's often down to the child of a deaf patient to interpret. Until you go through these battles yourself, you probably don't realise how hearing-focused everyday life is. The doctor calling your name at a hospital appointment, health-and-safety announcements, live government announcements on TV, radio shows / podcasts and speaking events are just a few things that deaf people cannot access.

Humans are social beings. We like to communicate with each other, and that interaction doesn't have to be audible. Also, in case you were wondering, deaf people can still party! BSL interpreter Chelsea Fields describes going out dancing with her deaf friends: 'If we were near the speakers they could feel the vibrations, and if not they would look around and see what rhythm others were moving to (slow or fast, etc.) and they would mimic those movements.' Yes, even though there are sound barriers, we still like to have a good time, and being deaf doesn't mean that needs to stop! We can still enjoy music, whether through vibrations or listening to the melody rather than the lyrics. As Rose Ayling-Ellis showed on *Strictly Come Dancing*, we don't have to hear the music in full to be able to dance and enjoy it.

It's important to remember that many people are experiencing the same accessibility challenges as you are. As I've mentioned, 12 million people in the UK have some form of hearing loss or deafness. Blogger Bethan Harvey advises: 'Never ever be afraid to reach out and ask for help. Ask all the questions, speak your worries and concerns – make sure you reach out, as there is no such thing as a silly question.' Many members of the deaf community are happy to offer advice. And remember that you can get support from family, friends, charities and your GP too. You can also check out the Resources section of this book.

Concentration fatigue

'Tiredness and fatigue are common problems for deaf children. They often have to concentrate harder to follow conversations, whether in speech or signed. Understanding that this fatigue is related to deafness is an important first step,' explains NDCS.

However, concentration fatigue doesn't just affect deaf children. Blogger Bethan Harvey explains that:

> Deafness and hearing loss affects your energy levels, with something known as listen fatigue. This comes from increased focus and concentration, whether this is following a conversation or being extra-alert to your surroundings. It is physically and mentally exhausting to keep up and follow along with hearing people. Our brains are constantly having to try to piece things together. Someone might say 'Liverpool'. I would maybe get L-v-p-o-l and I then have to try to piece together what words or letters fit to make what's been said make sense.

Concentration fatigue really affects me and other deaf people. I know if I have an event to attend where there will be lots of people and background noise, and I will have to lip-read in difficult surroundings (group scenarios or low lighting), I will be very tired the next day and will be unable to complete my usual amount of work. And I don't just mean that social events are tricky; in my industry there are a lot of work events in similar surroundings too.

I was lucky enough to be a judge recently for the Royal Television Society awards. The awards evening was a fabulous, star-studded occasion and I wore full sequins – yes, even my shoes were sequinned. It was a brilliant night, and I spent it celebrating TV talent, seeing old friends, and smiling at TV commissioners in the hope they will one day give me my own show. It was of course noisy, despite being in a venue that wasn't too bad acoustically. There were lots of soft furnishings to soak up the sound, but with a few hundred people chatting, a sit-down meal, music and an awards show being presented, there was a lot going on. We were at round tables. While this makes it easier to lip-read the people on either side of you, the table centrepieces and bottles of wine make lip-reading across the table harder. It was an evening event so the lighting was low, and there were lots of new people to meet, which meant getting used to lip-reading new people with different lip and speech patterns. Also, when there is background noise people automatically want to talk into your ear to help you hear them, but this doesn't help me because I need to see their mouth – and I don't need any more shouting in my ears, thanks!

The RTS were, in fact, very considerate: they asked if there was anything I needed access-wise before the event, and seemed committed to making things easier for me. Full disclosure: there was a BSL interpreter, and I didn't email them a full list of requirements because it felt like kicking up a fuss, and I was just excited to be part of the whole thing.

You might ask why I go to these events if I find them so tiring, but if I didn't go to these things, I'd never leave the house! It's important to say here that I do have fun at these events: the RTS awards was one of my best nights of the year and I have always loved dressing up, meeting new people and having interesting discussions with them – that's the joy of socialising, and I'm a very sociable person. However, I know that I will have a concentration fatigue hangover, so I might not say yes to quite as many events, and I'll make sure I have time to recover the next day.

So if you see me or another deaf person at an event, or if you want to organise an event that deaf people will be attending, what can you do to help? Here are some top tips.

- Make it as easy as possible for us to lip-read you.
- Have captioned *and* BSL interpreted performances/announcements.
- Organise events in rooms with acoustic panelling (which absorbs sound) or soft furnishings.
- Have quieter break-out spaces for respite.
- Have some tables with better lighting to put lip-readers on (not sitting deaf people next to music speakers also helps).
- Be aware of noise levels, and turn music down if it's too loud.
- Create seating spaces with curtains like a little boudoir. These seating spaces can create a pocket of quieter space.
- Outdoor events (where there are no walls to bounce sound off) are good too.

There you are – some great tips for any friends who want to organise a surprise birthday party for me!

And it's not just in-person events: even Zoom and FaceTime calls can be tiring due to having to constantly lip-read and concentrate on hearing what other people are saying. Using platforms with live captioning/subtitles can help, and a lot of deaf people told me that Google Meet is best for this.

Concentration fatigue is also something I had to come to terms with as part of my career as a performer. While I am capable of being a deaf stand-up comedian, the concentration fatigue associated with gigging three or four nights a week was huge and affected my daytime jobs (writing, radio and acting). And

I'm not alone. Charlotte Hyde explains: 'You will be more tired than you ever have been. Concentration fatigue is awful. Therefore, it's so important that you communicate when you're struggling.'

I was definitely struggling. My anxiety was getting worse, I was so tired and I felt dangerously close to burnout, trying to keep up with everything. I took the decision to stop performing stand-up live to protect my mental health and to alleviate some of the concentration fatigue I was experiencing. I realised that of all the aspects of my career, live stand-up tended to be the loudest, darkest and most overwhelming environment. It's not being on stage that was trying, as I'd have a mic then and I'd be the only one talking. No, it was the travelling to and from the gig, the background noise in the venues before and afterwards, poor lighting (because people laugh more in the dark), backstage areas with bad acoustics, meeting groups of tense people thinking about their own acts rather than keeping their mouths clear (which is fair enough if you're about to perform). While live comedy is wonderful and should be funded and supported, I found it was becoming more and more tiring for me, and this affected my mental health. Luckily, book writing is a pretty quiet endeavour (apart from when my dog Custard tries to get my attention), and radio and acting generally take place in sound-controlled environments, so I was able to continue being creative in those ways. I guess I'm still amusing, so I still call myself a comedian. There will always be a part of me that misses the buzz of a live gig, but I have to say it's been a huge relief since I stopped. The comedian in me wants to say it's a huge relief for my audiences as well, but the self-advocate in me wants you to know that I was actually pretty good (winning awards and selling out venues, don't you know).

I can totally empathise with anyone who feels they need to reduce their working hours or even quit their job due to a lack of accessibility. I hope this is becoming less and less common, but I understand how frustrating this can feel.

Sound sensitivity (hyperacusis)

So, you're deaf. That means everything you hear is muffled, right? Well, not exactly. Some people, like me – and it can be more common among those with noise-induced hearing loss and tinnitus – have heightened sensitivity to certain noises. So while I may not be able to make out everything you are saying in a noisy restaurant, someone chewing next to me can be so loud it's almost painful. The same is true of clinking glasses in a pub, a dog barking, or someone laughing at a certain pitch. These sounds will grab my attention and suddenly become all I can hear, which can be very distracting! I sometimes feel like the dog in the film *Up*, who will be mid-conversation (yes, the dog speaks in the film; it's not really a spoiler) then he will spot something out of the corner of his eye and shout 'Squirrel!' I guess my version is 'horrible sound!' but maybe I'll call them squirrels from now on. Of course, I don't shout 'Squirrel!' in a busy restaurant, but my attention has been diverted, and I often worry that people think I'm bored with talking to them or not engaged in the conversation as I seem distracted. (There is an upside, though: I guess it makes playing it cool on dates a lot easier . . .)

The NHS website explains: 'Hyperacusis is when every-day sounds seem much louder than they should. Treatment can help. See a GP if you think you have hyperacusis.'[46] I have never seen a GP about my hyperacusis; I've had other things on my list to deal with, such as tinnitus, hearing loss and hearing aids, as well as all the reproductive medical fun of being a woman. However, there are ways you can manage the condition.

Hyperacusis can be brought on by other conditions, such as head injuries, which can be treatable. If there's no clear cause, you may be offered treatment to help make you less sensitive to everyday sounds. This could involve:

- Sound therapy to get you used to everyday sounds again, and may involve wearing ear pieces that make white noise.
- Cognitive behavioural therapy (CBT) to change the way you think about your hyperacusis and reduce anxiety.[47]

The impact of your deaf experience on your friends and loved ones

I'm lucky enough to have a mum with hearing aids, which meant that my family had some idea of what it would be like when I got a hearing aid too. I also had someone to turn to with any questions, which made the process easier and less lonely. However, my mum is of a generation that believed being deaf wasn't something to be open or proud about, so she didn't have any connections with the wider deaf community – or much awareness of available support. In fact, I was the one who told my mum about Disabled Persons Railcards and the Access to Work grant, and encouraged her to see how more advanced hearing aids could be better for her. So we can positively educate and support friends and loved ones with their knowledge about the deaf world, hearing loss and deaf awareness. I am now someone people turn to if they discover they have hearing loss or want to understand how hearing aids might help them.

Finding out that you are deaf may shock those who have no experience of hearing loss or deafness. In her book *Hearing Happiness: Deafness Cures in History*, Jaipreet Virdi describes being taken to temples by her Sikh relatives to be prayed over, and given herbs and tinctures to try and 'cure' her. She describes her mother as 'convinced my deafness was divine punishment for her failings as a parent'.[48] She goes on to say: 'My father blamed my mother. My mother blamed the doctor . . . And I blamed myself: I must have done something naughty to deserve this.' As Jaipreet goes on to explain in her book, being deaf is absolutely *not* a punishment or disease or bad karma. However, some families react negatively, due to social or religious stigma around deafness and other disabilities. Activist Charlotte Hyde says:

> I remember worrying about how my mum felt about my diagnosis. I think she mourned for the hearing child she thought I would be, as well as worried about my future. It's not something I blame her for at all – I think it's a natural parental instinct. One thing I do regret is how responsible I felt for how my family felt about my deafness.

Charlotte is correct that her family's reaction isn't their fault; it can be due to their upbringing and lots of outside factors. Nonetheless, it can be incredibly damaging to a deaf individual. It is important to say here that if you are deaf, there is nothing 'wrong' with you. You are not being punished – by a god or by anyone else. Being deaf is not your 'fault'. You don't have a disease – and please don't waste time looking for a cure. You are wonderful, unique and exactly the way you are supposed to be for your journey through this world. You will have a gorgeous life with gorgeous people – please don't believe anyone who tells you otherwise.

Loved ones worry about you because they care, but it can be exhausting to calm the fears of those around you, while also educating yourself and processing your experiences. Setting up boundaries can be really useful to protect your own mental health. Rather than answering everyone's questions yourself, you could direct them to informative websites like RNID or NDCS. We're lucky to have such a wealth of deaf community-led resources and information available on the internet at the click of a button. Previous generations weren't so lucky in this respect, although I hear that being able to play outside and not have to lock your doors was nice.

You might go through this process with close family and friends and then have to repeat it with your wider circle of friends or any time you begin a new job and have to tell people you are deaf. Blogger Bethan Harvey says: 'There can be a lack of compassion, understanding and empathy. Many hearing people I've come across haven't known what to do or how to respond when finding out I'm deaf, and usually go silent on me. There is very much a division of them and us.'

Some people may react to news of your deafness with silence or awkwardness, and it's important to remember that this says far more about them than it does about you. Often it is a lack of education that leaves people feeling uncomfortable and not knowing what to say. You may be happy to help educate them, but remember that is not part of your job as a deaf person – it's up to them to educate themselves. Your workplace can help educate your colleagues with deaf awareness training (see Chapter 12 on work), which I believe all workplaces should provide, whether or not they have deaf members of staff.

Your family and friends will learn about the joys of being deaf over time. Amy Morton says the best thing about her deafness is 'being able to take my aids out when my kids are being loud or I need a break from noise if I've been exposed to it. I literally take them out and can still hear some sound, but not the intensity, and it's bliss!! I am the envy of my mum friends.'

I like to play music through my hearing aid if something is going on that I don't want to listen to but I still need to appear attentive.

Understanding and patience are important, both for you and those close to you, although that can be easier said than done. Keighley Miles from FDC explains: 'It's tiring having to try hard to understand what they are saying to me, and sometimes I just want no one to talk to me, then I feel guilty because I feel like I shouldn't feel like that about my children talking to me. I can get frustrated if I can't make out what they are saying, and they are the same.'

I have ended up in arguments with family members who get annoyed at having to repeat themselves, especially on a night out, for example, when they're more concerned with having fun. The other side of things is when I come across as rude by saying 'You're mumbling' or 'Why are you talking so quietly today?' because I'm frustrated that I have to ask someone to repeat themselves a lot. My poor sister, who has full hearing, has been on the receiving end of this. Sorry, Emily! I remember when she had temporary hearing loss due to a wax build-up, she moaned about not being able to hear things a lot, and I was secretly glad that she'd got to experience a little of what it can be like to be deaf! But that's the vindictive sister in me, I guess. However, lovely moments can come from being deaf too, as Keighley Miles explains:

My children know and understand I'm deaf 99 per cent of the time and we have great conversations. Instead of talking when we're doing stuff, we actually have to stop what we're doing and give the conversation our full attention. When they were younger they were always in the room I was in because I was worried if they called me I wouldn't hear, and I think this has deepened our relationship.

I remember going on a trip to Amsterdam for my birthday with my sister and my best friend, and we ended up in a very fun but very noisy bar. I wanted to be somewhere with a good atmosphere but the background noise was making it so difficult to hear anything, and the only place we could sit was along a bench, the three of us in a row, which – coupled with the mood lighting – made lip-reading pretty hard. After having a moment of feeling sorry for myself and annoyed at the hearing world, I opened a BSL app on my phone and started showing them signs. It became a fun game to see how far we could get in conversation without looking up a sign (luckily they both knew some basic sign language). Suddenly we were all in the same boat, using facial expressions and gestures to communicate, and we had a really fun night. Charlotte Hyde explains:

It can be tricky in bars and loud venues, as I tire so easily and grow irritable. I often end up scrolling on my phone because it's so difficult for me to involve myself in the conversation. My friends are brilliant and will always check in with me on noise levels, but I've often said yes to going to places that are too loud for me because I didn't want to let everyone else down.

I can totally relate to this feeling of not wanting to disappoint friends who want to go to really trendy loud bars. It takes confidence to tell strangers about your communication needs, and sometimes it takes even more confidence to reinforce that with friends. There are some days when I don't want to have to be confident, self-advocate, and feel like the problem friend, so I zone out of the conversation, scroll on my phone, or even go home. I think it's important to remember that your friend wants to hang out with you: I'm sure they would much rather talk to you than stand in a loud bar, and you can always find a compromise. I have never regretted standing up for myself and my needs – but I have regretted not saying something and having a terrible night just because I didn't want to cause a fuss.

Deaf people are noisy

'There is a misconception in the hearing world that deaf people are quiet,' Sara Novic writes in her novel *True Biz*.[49] If you think about it, it is only your perception of sound that indicates when you are being 'too loud' or 'noisy', so people with profound deafness can be some of the noisiest people you will ever meet!

Keighley Miles reveals: 'Being deaf, I don't know how quiet/ loud I'm talking. I used to call the children and they would say "we didn't hear you" or "wow, why are you so loud?"' Comedian Angela Barnes explains, 'I can't hear my own voice, so I have a problem with regulating it because I can't hear it.'

This is something I can relate to. When I am at a speaking event using a microphone, I like to be able to hear my voice clearly through the mic, although you don't always get a good indicator of what sound the audience are hearing as the speakers are so often facing away from the performer. Many times I have played a game of dancing sound levels, as the sound technician turns my microphone down as they think I am speaking too loudly but then I can't hear myself clearly so I speak louder into the mic so I can hear myself, so they turn it down even more and so on until I am essentially shouting at the audience without the need for any amplification. Now, to avoid this dance, I am always open with the sound technician about my deafness and the fact I like to be able to hear my voice. This means they can turn the speakers a little more in my direction so I can hear myself better.

I realise that not everyone speaks using a microphone (everyone should get a chance to, though!), but this also applies to everyday life. If you can't hear yourself in a noisy environment, you might speak more loudly until you *can* hear yourself, and not realise that you are shouting at your friends. This volume control can be tricky when you're deaf, and your family and friends might notice this as a symptom of hearing loss.

People who use BSL aren't always quiet either, and will often use vocal sounds as part of their expression of emotions, alongside BSL. BSL is an emotive language as well as a physical one, so there may be sounds of hand-slapping if someone is signing angrily or enthusiastically. Deaf people love to laugh too, and express this vocally, as Sara Novic writes: 'Her mother laughed, a deep-gullet sound totally uninfluenced by what the world decided laughter should be.'[50] Plus there's tons of chair scraping, plate clinking, door slamming and all the usual sounds of everyday life.

Dogs

Yep, my dog Custard isn't mentioned enough in this book so far. There is actually a relevant reason for this section, though. Amy Morton tells a cautionary tale: 'A word of warning to all hearing-aid users!! Dogs eat hearing aids! Do be careful when leaving them around . . . Choki [the dog] found my hearing aid and had a good munch on it, including the ear mould, which I think was the bit that had hooked him in – the smell of the wax.' (Yes, I asked, and yes, the ear mould came out in Choki's poo, but Amy had already got a new hearing aid – phew!)

In fact, Custard has also tried to eat my hearing aid. She's managed to chew up the tubing and earbud twice now. The first time she really got stuck in, and my silver Phonak Audeo hearing aid still has a miniature dachshund-sized tooth indent on one side. Luckily, it still works and I could easily replace the tubing, but be warned. Always leave your hearing aids out of reach of any pets.

Dogs can also help us. Charity Hearing Dogs (www.hearing dogs.org.uk) provide dogs to support deaf people in everyday life. People with severe and profound deafness can apply via their website.

Deaf people can seem rude

Sometimes people think I am rude, but a lot of the time this is just because I can't hear things. I might not reply to something they have said, simply because I didn't hear it or understand the part of it that was a question, so I'm not aware that they need a response. Also, rather than smiling at a social occasion I might look stern (or slightly constipated) because I'm concentrating so hard on hearing, so sometimes people might assume I'm not having a good time.

Keighley Miles explains what happened when her eldest hearing child started school:

> I realised he did stuff that was considered rude or annoying, but which to us as a family was normal, like tapping me to get my attention, or pushing my face to look at his face. [He] thought he had to do this with all adults, so we had to explain he wasn't being rude. All deaf families have this issue. There are template letters you can print off to explain to the teachers, as many haven't had any experience of teaching deaf children or CODAs [children of deaf adults].

Waving to get someone's attention, rather than using their name, can be seen as rude in the hearing world. In the deaf community it's much easier, but many hearing people aren't aware of this and might react negatively to it. In addition, Clare-Louise English reveals:

> I lip-read and take in people's body language, though weirdly I don't tend to pick up on people's subtext. It's been pointed out to me that perhaps [as] all my focus is going on understanding what *is* being said that I don't have the capacity to spare to understand what people *aren't* saying! That makes sense to me. I like people who are direct.

This can also be true when communicating in written English with people who use BSL. As BSL has a different structure to

English, it is best to be clear and direct in your use of language when emailing someone who uses BSL. If you receive an email from a deaf person, bear in mind that English may not be their first language, and don't read too much into how short or to-the-point their email might be. A deaf person might send a thank-you email simply saying 'thank you', whereas I might send a thank-you email reading, 'Hi Rose, I just wanted to drop you a note to say thank you so, so much for reading my new book, *Living with hearing loss and deafness*. It honestly means so much that you would take time out of your busy schedule to read my words, and I am so appreciative. It has honestly made my day. Thank you again, Sam.'

Safety

I was at a launch party for a new TV show recently. I know – the glamour! I got the last train home, which was considerably less glamorous than the event. However, my usual late-night taxi ride from the station to my door, to avoid walking home alone in the dark, was impossible due to the fact there were absolutely no taxis in my area of Kent. Perhaps everyone in the UK was enjoying a late-night tour of the garden of England . . . Instead, I walked home at 1 a.m. through poorly lit residential areas, with only scavenging foxes for company. Any woman will know that it can be scary walking home alone during the day, let alone in the dark, and my deafness can make this an even scarier prospect.

I've never been a huge fan of the dark. When I was younger I would leave the hallway light on and my bedroom door ajar so I always had the welcoming glow of safety at the edge of my vision. At sleepovers at my friends' houses I would ask if they could leave the bathroom light on, just so I knew where it was if I woke up in the night. I'm not sure where my fear of the dark came from, but not being able to see what was in my room when I was at my most vulnerable, in those moments before sleep, really bothered me. If you add not being able to hear to this equation, the fear multiplies. As a deaf adult I wouldn't say I am necessarily *scared* of the dark, but I am definitely not comfortable in it. On that 1 a.m. walk home, I imagined all the awful humans who could be hiding around dark corners, watching me from slow-moving cars, or running up behind me. I love my hearing aid because it amplifies the sounds around me, but I still worry that I wouldn't hear someone creeping up behind me on an unlit street. I take out my hearing aids each night to sleep and charge them, and so then I'd be even less likely to hear an intruder creeping up the stairs. I feel more vulnerable as a deaf woman because I don't have hearing to warn me of an intruder.

So what can help make deaf people feel more secure at home? Doorbell cameras and video cameras for your home that link to your phone or Alexa, like the Ring doorbells and devices mentioned in Chapter 9, can help you feel safe in your home. You get a notification if the cameras detect any motion, and they can record video too, which can help the police catch and charge perpetrators. The new 999 BSL app for contacting the emergency services if you use BSL (see Chapter 9) is also really useful to have on your phone.

Of course, you should also follow all the usual safety tips: try to avoid walking home late alone; if you have to, walk in well-lit areas; call or FaceTime a friend on the way; share your live location with a friend on your journey home; text a friend to let them know you have arrived home safely.

It's not just walking home in the dark that can be tricky for deaf people. Comedian Angela Barnes says: 'I wonder how I haven't died just walking in front of a car, because I can't hear cars coming.' This is a big worry at the beginning of your deaf journey, especially if you have hearing loss later in life. However, you will learn to compensate for this by developing incredible peripheral vision. A 2017 study[51] found that deaf people develop an enhanced level of visual perception, which is why many deaf people are excellent drivers. Having to be aware of your surroundings visually, as you can't rely on sounds, can help you with crossing the road, driving, dancing – basically any physical activity where you have to navigate space. These skills will develop over time and can be improved by lip-reading and BSL classes, which also teach you to be more aware of visual cues.

Acoustically pleasant surroundings

Finding a quiet spot, or at least a place with minimal background noise, can make you feel more comfortable meeting friends socially. Distinguishing voices from background noise can be incredibly difficult for those with hearing loss. My top tip to find your nearest quiet spot is to use the SoundPrint app, which uses crowdsourced reviews and decibel ratings for cafes, bars and restaurants in your area.

The website quietliving.co.uk is also an excellent resource if you are looking for quiet areas in the UK, or tips to reduce sound in your home or office/venue. If you get to know a local business owner, you could always advise them on ways to make their venue quieter, or perhaps they could even start something like 'Quiet Tuesdays', where every Tuesday they don't play background music or use loud machinery/coffee machines. You can pitch it as a marketing idea that will draw in a crowd of people who prefer less noisy surroundings.

DeafSpace

The DeafSpace project was founded in 2005 by architect Hansel Bauman and with the ASL Deaf Studies Department at Gallaudet University in Washington, DC. Its aim was to develop DeafSpace guidelines for designing spaces for deaf people. The guidelines cover things like acoustics, space, light, colour and sensory reach.

To find out more, visit the Gallaudet website, which, among other things, explains:

> When deaf people get together, they often work together to rearrange the furniture into a 'conversation circle' to allow clear sightlines so everyone can participate in the visual conversation. Gatherings usually start with participants adjusting window shades, lighting, and seating to optimise conditions for visual communication that minimise eye strain . . . These practical acts of making a DeafSpace are long-held cultural traditions.[52]

It is very important that environments like schools and offices are acoustically pleasant for deaf and hearing people alike. Teacher Victoria Sylvester says: 'We have fabric boards on walls and low ceilings to absorb sound to make sounds much clearer for our students' – and this is something that all working environments can implement. 'If less than 50 per cent of your ceiling and less than 20–30 per cent of your walls are not covered with sound-absorbing materials, then your venue is more likely to experience noise issues,' explains the SoundPrint app website.[53]

Here are some top tips for making your venue / office acoustically pleasant:

- Turn down background music (especially if the place is busy).
- Move loud machinery – e.g. coffee machines/blenders – so they are not near seating areas.
- Add soft furnishings to absorb sound. Cushions and curtains can do wonders, as well as making your space more comfy!
- Add carpets to absorb sound – and retain heat.
- Segment the seating areas by using fencing/curtains/plants/walls to help contain the noise.
- Add acoustic panels to large echoey spaces. These panels can be used on the floor, ceiling or walls. All acoustic panels should comply with the noise reduction laws and fire regulations in your country.
- Add sound-absorbing artworks (there are lots on Etsy) that not only reduce sound levels but are also aesthetically pleasing.
- Plus, train your staff to be deaf aware, of course!

You can design the interior, using carpets, soft furnishings and acoustic panels (these are widely available online and in DIY stores). You can even create your own acoustic panels by making a wooden rectangular structure, filling it with a dense insulation/absorption panel (this looks like a type of foam) then covering the whole thing with your choice of fabric, which you can staple to the panel. You can buy a roll of insulation material for around £25 online, and fibreglass mesh reinforced insulation membrane costs around the same. Remember, you will need to fireproof these too.

So there you go, there are lots of ways to make your space more acoustically pleasant for deaf people. You could recycle cushions and soft furnishings from your house, charity shops or second-hand retailers if you are worried about cost. Also remember that workplaces have a legal obligation to make reasonable adjustments for their employees. While they might not consent to knocking down the office and rebuilding it with noise reduction in mind, they should agree to acoustic panels, cushions and segmented areas at least. That sounds like a reasonable adjustment to me.

Experiences of being deaf across the world

Things definitely need to improve for the deaf community in the UK, but it's also good to keep up to date with what is going on in the rest of the world. There's been a huge surge in exposure for American Sign Language (ASL) due to the success of the film *CODA*, made by an American team. This celebration of ASL means that brands and lifestyle labels are responding by including ASL signs on their clothing/stationery, etc., raising awareness of sign language.

A lot of this filters through to the UK market. ASL uses a one-handed sign alphabet, and that's a useful way to distinguish whether a product has a BSL (two-handed alphabet) or ASL sign on it. You could always learn BSL too! Of course, ASL signs aren't relevant to BSL speakers, so you'd probably want to buy a product from a deaf brand based in the UK, like

Deaf Identity, which makes clothes and accessories with BSL signs on them.

While deaf awareness is increasing in the UK, Europe and America, it is also important to know how deaf people are being treated across the world. Unfortunately, the news isn't always good. The World Federation of the Deaf states:

> In some countries, deaf people face discrimination and are unable to marry, inherit property, vote, or become elected, become a jury member or reproduce children. Deaf people are often deprived from participation in the political life due to poor accessibility, and lack of information in sign language on political affairs debates and questions. Because they are unequally treated in this respect they are unable to make informed choices and many become politically inactive.[54]

This is shocking to read, and emphasises the importance of deaf awareness and supporting deaf brands/businesses/spokespeople from across the world. We still have a lot of work to do.

Protecting your residual hearing

Being aware of damaging sound levels can be really useful to protect the hearing you do have. As you know, noise pollution can affect your hearing over time – I know I have become acutely aware of sound levels since I got my hearing aid. As mentioned before, you can download a decibel meter on your phone as an app and use it to measure sound levels in noisy environments. Remember, anything above 85 decibels for a prolonged period of time is proven to be damaging. Many of us try to avoid noisy environments, but try not to let this stop you leaving your house and meeting people.

I have experienced periods of anxiety where I have not wanted to venture outside and the idea of wearing my 'hearing mask' becomes too much. I have retreated to my safe space, my home, which I can control, and it has been hard to push myself back out into the world again. For me, having supportive family and friends made me take tentative steps back into the world – and I am so glad I did. By putting boundaries in place for myself and being open and honest about my communication needs, I have found it much more manageable to be out in public. A social night out can be really fun, but I will be very tired afterwards and, as I mentioned before, will sometimes need a couple of days to recover (from the sound, not even the alcohol!). Now that I am aware of this, I can be mindful of my schedule and make sure I give myself the time I need in between those noisy environments. If you are currently avoiding meeting up with friends because of sound levels and listening fatigue, then I encourage you to take the leap and go out. The mental health benefits of seeing your friends are just as important.

Why not use the SoundPrint app to discover quiet venues to meet friends for drinks? Perhaps you can meet for lunch rather than dinner, as venues tend to be quieter during the day. Or meet a friend for a walk in a location you know, and grab a coffee to take with you. Being honest really helps. Saying some-thing like 'I find coffee shops really overwhelming with my hearing aids – would you mind ordering the coffees if I give you the cash?' can not only help you avoid an environment that might make you feel uncomfortable, but will also help your friend understand how they can help you. Good friends will be more than happy to help.

Wearing ear defenders or earplugs in loud environments is also a good idea, and could provide you with some peace of mind. I was provided with an attenuator for a theatre job I was doing recently. Attenuators reduce the level of sound to a non-damaging level rather than completely blocking the ear. My attenuator was created with an ear mould, so it's person-alised to fit my ear and lets some sound through. I keep my attenuator in my purse so I can use it in my non-hearing-aid ear whenever things get too noisy. Modern hearing aids should also be able to adjust to environments so that they are not letting a damaging level of noise into your ears. You can speak to your audiologist about having a 'night-out setting', which you can switch your hearing aid to in environments with a lot of loud background noise.

Educating others

Constantly having to educate others about your deafness can be a tiring task. (I do realise the irony of that sentence written in a book that hopes to educate others!) Basically, I have written this book so I can hand it to people who have questions about being deaf or who want me to tell them what it's like to be deaf.

Person: 'Sam, what is it really like being deaf?'

Sam: (Hands person a copy of this book.) 'Read this.'

Any other deaf people reading this are welcome to do this too if you think it will help. Having said that, while I get tired of being a teacher to hearing people, I always love meeting deaf people or people who are beginning their deaf journey. Nothing makes me happier than answering questions from someone who has just found out they need a hearing aid, or thinks they have hearing loss and doesn't know what to do next. But giving advice isn't my full-time job. While I love to help, at some point I need to get on with living and earning money to pay for – you know, food and things. Sometimes it can be difficult to stop educating or trying to help because of feelings of guilt or the idea that you are being selfish by not supporting others. However, Actor David Bower explains: 'It's just not humanly possible to teach "deaf awareness" to everybody 24/7, and sometimes you have to cut your losses in order to quickly move on. Maybe that's part of self-preservation.'

Boundaries are important to help us live our lives and to avoid becoming completely defined by our disabilities. As Rose Ayling-Ellis said in her speech at the Edinburgh TV Festival in 2022, 'disabled people shouldn't be responsible for curing non-disabled people of their ignorance'.[55]

Charlotte Hyde advises: 'There is a difference between being able to hear and being able to understand. You could hear that someone is speaking to you and not understand a word they are saying. This is a helpful distinction to keep in mind when explaining your deafness to others. Also remember that your audiogram [the hearing graph you are given after an audiologist appointment, which charts your hearing level] is a reflection of your hearing in an artificial environment and will not accurately reflect your hearing in real-life situations.' Hearing people tend to be very interested in your level of deafness, and will ask you how deaf you are. This is invasive and irrelevant; you never need to disclose this information if you don't want to. In fact, David Bower says: 'Preserving one's sanity can mean knowing when it's time to let go, and that isn't always the easiest thing to do.' Letting go of the idea that you must educate the hearing world, or fight every battle, or change the accessibility in your workplace for everyone, not just yourself, is hard – but sometimes very necessary. Remember, you can always ask others, deaf and hearing alike, as well as organisations to help you.

Hearing loss and deafness: the positives

Mark Atkinson states: 'We need to dismantle the idea that hearing loss means the end of life as you know it.' Hearing loss was the beginning for me in so many ways. It has made me a more empathetic human, more expressive and compassionate. It has been the reason I started writing books. It has given me the passion to speak confidently as myself, not just telling jokes, and has given me a reason to get behind something. I have started doing more charity work, which is incredibly rewarding and fun. I've met some awesome new friends and been exposed to incredible events, people and experiences. I've spoken to large corporations and TV and radio journalists to raise deaf awareness. I've been part of discussions at the House of Commons. I have interviewed deaf actors and film crews and met Oscar award-winner Marlee Matlin and model and Deaf activist Nyle DiMarco. (Now I feel like I'm showing off, but you get the idea. None of these things would have happened if I wasn't deaf.)

While I am aware that I have a level of privilege as a white woman who works in the media, I also think that going on a journey to feel pride in my deafness and talking openly about it has opened doors by encouraging others to address accessibility and awareness. If you speak openly to your boss about being deaf, maybe your workplace could pay you to be a deaf advocacy officer or offer extra support to further your career there. Finding a local deaf community might lead to new friendships and learning new skills. Taking a BSL class could mean you meet the next love of your life! You will never know unless you give it a go.

RNID advocacy officer Annie Harris agrees:

> Deafness does not always have to be a bad thing. I wish people could see the positives from it, and understand why we wear our deafness with pride. I think it's important for doctors to be more positive when they provide the diagnosis to parents, simply by starting with 'your baby is deaf' rather than saying 'I'm so sorry, your baby is suffering from hearing loss.' Then follow this up with information about sign language, positive deaf role models, as well as medical options. If parent and child have a good beginning from the start, the child will grow up feeling happy with a good supportive network.

One thing many deaf people agree on is that they love the ability to switch off from sound completely. Blogger Bethan Harvey says: 'I've always slept on my left "good ear", so I literally cannot hear anything. I've always loved being able to sleep through anything and everything that would typically wake someone, such as thunderstorms. I'm totally oblivious.'

I agree: I love taking off my hearing aid after a busy day out and about. It's akin to getting into a hot bath or taking off your bra when you walk in the door. The relief!

Actor David Bower says: 'I have felt that the Deaf experience has been a strength for me, in that I believe it offers potentially unique ways of perceiving existence and to strike out from the herd and to forge an authentic path.'

This is true for many of the people I have interviewed for this book, who have created new businesses or careers inspired by their deaf experience. Annie Harris explains:

I am so lucky to be in a position where I can create meaningful change for the community. I love going to deaf theatres, or watching deaf films, or going to deaf events – all to experience the feeling of freedom where there are no barriers to communication. Only last week at a deaf event, I spotted someone talking about me in sign (saying lovely things) across a busy field. How amazing is that? When I cannot access conversation every day, day in and out, that moment is even more magical.

This is also true for Bethan Harvey:

I cannot forget the incredible opportunities that I've had, which I would not have had if I wasn't deaf, including starting my blog to raise awareness of deafness, TV and radio interviews, newspaper and magazine articles, winning a Rotary Young Citizen of the Year award, volunteering, and being involved with some amazing deaf charities, such as Families of Deaf Children Essex (FDC), Microtia UK and Essex Deaf Children's Society, being able to help and support the next generation of deaf children – and of course the incredible opportunity of being interviewed for books such as this one. I honestly love being deaf – I wouldn't change it for anything.

Chapter 12
Working with hearing loss

RNID says that 'if you're deaf or have hearing loss, your employer has a duty to make adjustments so you're not put at a disadvantage'. Those are your rights as an employee in the UK, under the Equality Act 2010: please remember that there are laws to protect you at work.

RNID lists 'reasonable adjustments' as:

- adjusting the layout of a meeting room and using good lighting to help everybody see each other clearly (important for lip-reading)
- modifying a job to take your needs into account
- moving you to an office with good acoustics where sound is transmitted well
- providing communication support[56] for meetings, such as speech-to-text reporters
- installing equipment,[57] such as amplified telephones or flashing-light fire alarms
- providing a portable hearing loop for you to use during a training course away from the office
- giving you time off work for your audiology appointments[58]

Their website states that:

> If your hearing loss is relatively minor and it doesn't affect your day-to-day life, it's unlikely that you'll be protected by the Equality Act. But if your hearing loss has a substantial effect on your ability to carry out normal day-to-day activities, you'll be protected. If you are covered by the Act, you'll also be protected against discrimination (including the failure to make reasonable adjustments), harassment and victimisation.

I would argue that all hearing loss affects your day-to-day life, as hearing things is a day-to-day activity. In the workplace, employers also have regulations they are obliged to meet by law when it comes to working in noisy environments, and your employer should provide you with hearing protection if this is the case. You can check the sound levels in your workplace by downloading a decibel meter on your mobile.

It is shocking that Deaf Unity states that 'a deaf or hard-of-hearing person is 4 times more likely to be unemployed than a hearing person'.[59] This is unacceptable and needs to be addressed by society. Blogger Bethan Harvey reveals: 'I've had both positive and negative experiences relating to my deafness in the workplace. Some workplaces have been great about it . . . others, not so much.' And Annie Harris, RNID advocacy officer, told me about a previous job: 'I experienced discrimination to an extent that I had to leave, because I had no support to accommodate my deafness. They made me feel I was stupid and not good at my job.' Author and Deaf historian Kathleen L. Brockway remembers: 'Deaf employees often faced discrimination at work. Often they were the last people to know what was going on in the workplace. I worked in the hearing world and have experienced so many roadblocks.' However, when the right access is put in place for us, deaf people can thrive. BSL teacher and SignSong performer Fletch@ explains: 'I have an interpreter who assists me for office work, telephone calls and guidance with my sign songs so that I ensure I remain on time with the music.'

Is discrimination in the workplace down to the fact that we don't know enough about our rights? How would you know about the Equality Act 2010 and what it means unless you'd been taught about it at school, informed when you have your audiology appointments, or told about it by your employer? It is important we don't put the blame on deaf people ourselves. Yes, I have done a trolley-load of research for this book, but who has time to do that while trying to get a job, pay for hearing assistance devices, and deal with the mental health issues that come along with being deaf?

It is important that we all know our rights (hopefully this book will help with that) – but it's also important for employers to know them too – and to act on them. Hearing people can be excellent allies in making sure that deaf people in the workplace get the support we need. Here are some suggestions of ways to support deaf people at work:

- 'Shall we send the presentation to Samantha in advance so she can read through it now, and then she can focus on lip-reading during the presentation?'
- 'Oh, we need to book a BSL interpreter for that meeting.'
- 'Can we use meeting room five as it is quieter?'

- 'Let's ask Sam if there's anything she would like us to organise, communication-wise.'
- 'I'll reserve a seat for Sam at the front so she can lip-read.'
- 'I will let the visiting speaker know we have deaf colleagues so they will need to speak clearly, not cover their mouths, and wear a device around their neck.'

I could go on, but then the whole book would be a list of ally role-play, which should clearly be my next book. And it's not just about having allies. Stigma, hostile working environments, and employers not being aware of our rights all come into play, as paediatric nurse and deaf awareness advocate Asha explains:

Being Deaf in a healthcare setting has its own challenges as there are a lot of assumptions that deaf people cannot do certain things, such as listening to chest sounds with a stethoscope. Working in a hospital is not the best environment to work in due to the poor acoustics and the noisy environment. I have come across people who have questioned why I am doing nursing if I cannot hear; if anything, this pushes me even further to achieve what I want in my career.

Charlotte Hyde also experienced audist (audism is the belief that being able to hear makes you superior to someone who is deaf) reactions:

When I went back to my retail job, I had one too many customers congratulating me for 'doing so well' and telling me it was fantastic that I 'actually had a job' – with the implication that other deaf people don't work. Each instance was – quite frankly – patronising, and the insinuation that other deaf people don't work was insulting to the entire deaf community.

So how do we fight prejudice and difficult environments? Perhaps we start even earlier, in educational environments. Schools can be the perfect starting point to make accessibility a priority and lead the way so that, from a young age, both deaf and hearing children see examples of effective accessible environments. Unfortunately this is not currently the case. While there are brilliant, hard-working teachers out there making a huge difference, due to government cuts in funding for education there are many issues that need addressing in our schools. However, access is a basic human right. If access is not prioritised in schools in the UK then we are not providing a fair education for all children, which is surely the core aim of our education system.

So if we reduce our expectations and simply hope for a good education for deaf children, equal to that of hearing children, is that being achieved? Can we confidently say that deaf children are getting the same education as hearing children? Especially in mainstream schools? In 2022 it was reported that deaf children received a whole GCSE grade lower overall than hearing children[60] – for the seventh year running! Seven years! That's a whole school education cycle. That's the whole time it took Harry Potter to discover he was a wizard, learn about magic and defeat Voldemort – and we can't even make schools accessible for deaf children.

Deaf blog Limping Chicken reported:

> The National Deaf Children's Society has called on the government to use its review into special educational needs and disabilities (SEND) to improve long-term support for deaf children, including an investment in more teachers of the deaf. Numbers of specialist staff have declined over the past decade, by 17 per cent . . . In a statement, a Department for Education spokesperson told the Limping Chicken: 'All children and young people, including those who are deaf or have a hearing impairment, should receive the support they need to succeed in their education. There is a legal requirement for qualified teachers to hold relevant mandatory qualifications when teaching classes of pupils who have a sensory impairment.'[61]

Please see Chapter 1 to find out what I think about the use of 'hearing impairment' here – and from the Department for Education, no less!

So charities are calling on the government to make changes – and the government seems to be blaming the situation on teachers?

This isn't a new thing either. Keighley Miles recalls: 'I dropped out of school, and even though I tried to get back into education, it never lasted because I always struggled to hear and I didn't know I could get support.'

Why isn't BSL taught in school just like French and Spanish and English are? I don't remember deaf history being part of my curriculum. When we learnt how the ear works in biology, we didn't go on to find out how hearing aids work with the ear to amplify sounds, or what happens to your hearing if your ear is damaged. Something has to change in the education system. We need to continue to support (for example, by funding, volunteering, sharing their messages, or supporting and amplifying their campaigns) charities like NDCS and RNID that are lobbying for change. We need to call out audism when we see it, and hold our local schools to account. This shouldn't be down to deaf people; it's down to us all.

Problems in the workplace: reporting colleagues

But what do you do if the people you work with *are* the problem? Charlotte says: 'I always remind myself that I don't have to put up with ignorance. I've had to go to higher-ups about colleagues before and, while it was awkward at the time, I don't regret it.' Although it may be hard in the moment, you have the right to work in a job and be treated fairly and respectfully. If someone else is having a negative impact on your work environment then that's their issue and not your fault in any way.

Deaf disability benefits advisor Jasper Williams says:

> I would always recommend keeping a record of any incident(s) so you have some form of evidence. Include when it happened, where, and what happened, if there were any witnesses, etc. If you feel comfortable doing so, you could talk to your manager about the incident. If nothing changes or if you are uncomfortable [speaking to your manager], raise a grievance. Your workplace will have a formal procedure, but it usually involves putting in writing what happened and what you

want resolved. Ask HR if you do not know the process. In your complaint, remind them of the law: the Equality Act 2010 protects disabled people from discrimination in the workplace. If your complaint is still is not resolved, seek legal advice. Your union, if you have joined one, may be able to help, and there are other places you can get free impartial advice from too, including:

1. Advisory, Conciliation and Arbitration Service (ACAS)
2. Equality Advisory Support Service (EASS)
3. Royal Association of the Deaf
4. Fry Legal
5. DID Law[62]
6. Disability Law Service

If you have access issues with the person you are getting legal advice from, direct them to the Law Society.[63]

Problems with employers

When we are looking at access to work, the big hurdle is often employers. Why is it only down to the deaf individual to know their rights in the workplace? Shouldn't that be the prerogative of the employer? Mark Atkinson, RNID chief exec, says:

The biggest issues we've found facing our (very diverse) communities are around inclusion and barriers to accessing many of the services and spaces hearing people take for granted. We know that many employers don't feel confident in recruiting and supporting candidates who are deaf, have hearing loss or tinnitus.

How can we change this? RNID and other organisations offer deaf awareness training for your workplace. This is useful not just for deaf employees, but also for customers. Louder than Words (the training arm of RNID) states on its website that: 'Research shows that more than 70 per cent of people who use hearing aids would choose a company with staff who are deaf aware over a company whose staff are not.' If you own a business, think of all those extra customers! What's especially great about paying a deaf charity to provide deaf awareness training is that your money is going towards all the good work the charity is doing as well as the service they are providing for you. The Inklusion Guide (set up to address accessibility in the publishing industry) says: 'It is imperative that you employ disabled staff. Listen to their experience and recommendations. However, it is important to note that disabled staff are not experts on disability, and it shouldn't be assumed that they are or that they should be expected to do an access role on top of their own work.'[64]

Asking your employees what help they might need is also an important, and often overlooked, way to support them. Arranging to meet them for a coffee, out of the office (in a quiet coffee shop!) for a chat about how they're getting on and how you can support them is so appreciated. As is cultivating an environment where your employees feel that they can open up to you about their hearing loss/deafness. Accessibility training can be a great way to open up these conversations. Having an Access Officer is important for all organisations. This should be a person with appropriate qualifications as well as lived experience.

Environments that hearing people take for granted can be incredibly unwelcoming for a deaf person. For example, blogger Bethan Harvey describes working for a fast-food chain: 'When working on the till there is an incredible amount of noise from customers chatting and eating, kids screaming and laughing in the play area, staff taking customers' orders, timers on fryers going off, kitchen staff talking, staff shouting orders to the kitchen . . .'

Employers can book a workplace assessment through places like Louder than Words for any deaf employees. The employee will speak to the assessor face to face. The follow-up report will 'outline cost-effective adjustments, such as improving the working environment, offering flexible working or providing assistive technology. Everyone is different so the recommendations will vary.'[65]

This is an excellent way to support your staff, but I know what you're thinking: 'Yes, Sam, but how much does it cost?' Well, having this type of training and assessment will ensure that you are fulfilling your duties as an employer under the Equality Act 2010. The Louder than Words website also states: 'The assessment report can be used to apply for the government's Access to Work funding.[66] This will help you cover the cost of purchasing equipment and support, ensuring increased productivity and improved job satisfaction.'

Funding

If you would like help at work, there are funds available, such as the Access to Work grant, to help pay for practical support and equipment. Through Access to Work, you can apply for:

- a grant to help pay for practical support with your work
- support with managing your mental health at work
- money to pay for communication support at job interviews[67]

This grant covers things like BSL interpreters and note-takers. The UK government website states:

Your workplace can include your home if you work from there some or all of the time. It does not matter how much you earn. If you get an Access to Work grant, it will not affect any other benefits you get and you will not have to pay it back. You or your employer may need to pay some costs up front and claim them back later.[68]

Deaf disability benefits advisor Jasper Williams says of the grant: 'It gives autonomy and independence back to D/deaf and hard-of-hearing people so they are able to work and attend interviews and reduce the anxiety/stress of working out how they can communicate.'

It is important to note that Access to Work does not pay for 'reasonable adjustments', as these are covered under the Equality Act and an employer is legally obliged to make them. You can also not apply for this fund to help with volunteer work. Self-employed work is eligible for support under the scheme. You can apply for the grant through the UK government website, and there is also a phone number, text service and BSL service. You can also request all correspondence to be done via email rather than phone call – hurrah!

To apply for the grant, you will have to suggest what support you need. Apart from an interpreter, you could list:

- a Zoom subscription (so you can lip-read during Zoom calls)
- transcription services
- computer software like VRS
- paid extra hours to review transcripts of live meetings/ presentations
- a personal assistant to review emails/transcripts/process text
- a speech-to-text reporter (people who live caption events)
- a radio aid (a microphone usually worn around a speaker's neck that transmits straight to your hearing aids)

You could even ask for hearing aids if you make a clear case for why you need a specific type that might not be available on the NHS, for example.

Jasper Williams advises:

> Think about all the different aspects of your work role and the exact support you need. For example, if there are phone calls you need to answer in your job, maybe you need a captioned phone or video relay service software such as SignLive or SignVideo. If you have remote meetings, maybe you need captioning software, lip-speakers [see p. 115], or BSL interpretation. If you need to process a lot of text in reports and you struggle with English, a communication support worker might be helpful. Do your research and have your lists ready before you apply.

Jasper also advises: 'You will be asked for likely three quotes for any support you ask for, so ask around and get this ready . . . If you are self-employed, you will be asked for a business plan – so if you don't have one yet, get writing!' As for other funding, Jasper says:

> D/deaf and hard-of-hearing people are eligible for applying for disability benefits, but this will vary greatly depending on their circumstances. They may be entitled to benefits such as Universal Credit, Employment and Support Allowance, and Personal Independence Payments. These are gateways to other support, such as free bus passes, Disabled Persons Railcards and +1 companions for events and theatre productions.

I use a Disabled Persons Railcard myself. It gives me a third off travel for myself and a companion (so they can tell me what all the station announcements are about). There are also access tickets available at theatres, which offer a discounted rate. If you are a lip-reader, for example, you can request a seat close to the front!

Will I lose my job because of my deafness?

One of my biggest worries when I was told I needed a hearing aid was my fear of losing my job. At the time I was acting in period dramas like *The Crown* and *Call the Midwife*, and I worried about having a modern hearing aid in a historical drama. There are so many reasons you can't get hired as an actor: you might be too tall/short, too brown-haired, too funny, you don't match the love interest, you're not available for the shoot dates, you've put on weight since they last saw you, you're 'too smiley' (yes, someone actually said this to me once). I was worried that 'she wears a hearing aid' was going to be one more thing on a long list of reasons not to hire me. Clare-Louise English of Hot Coals Productions had similar worries:

> My first thought was 'how can I be an actor now if I can't hear my cues on stage?' I was only fourteen but I already knew what I wanted to be, and where I wanted to go. I think that explains why I'm so fiercely protective of my career now, because I felt I'd almost lost it.

Sophie Stone was the first deaf actor to train at the Royal Academy of Dramatic Arts (RADA) (I auditioned back in the day, and only got through to the second round). Since her training, Sophie has become a role model for deaf actors and has performed in some incredible shows, including *Doctor Who*, *The Crown*, and an excellent *Casualty* storyline written by deaf screenwriter Charlie Swinbourne. She has also performed at the Globe and the National Theatre. I asked Sophie what it was like being the first deaf actor at RADA and she said:

> Tough. It was a real learning curve for all of us, staff and institution alike. We all learned a lot from each other. It was special being deemed worthy of being there, but getting in wasn't the be-all and end-all. It was where the work started. And access to the training was something that we worked hard to maintain. I was exhausted by the system but in many ways I was made stronger because of it. It made me able to ask for what I needed, but also to understand the 'business' I was graduating into. Not just for myself but for other Deaf

actors who wanted to train at drama schools but were turned away because of lack of access rather than a lack of talent. I knew I had work to do. Being a role model wasn't enough. The machine had to change. Since then, I've seen a change – the ball is finally rolling.

Seeing Sophie's incredible acting work and advocacy has definitely inspired me to open up about my deafness as an actor. I worked on a show called *Magic Mike Live* in London's West End, and for the first time was totally open and unapologetic about my hearing aid and deafness from the start. I had a great experience on that show, with the sound engineer making extra provisions for me and the producers providing hearing protection for the whole cast and sending me to an audiologist to create a special 'show' setting on my hearing aid for the change in sound environment. Also, yes – I met Channing Tatum, who directed the show. And yes, he does smell nice.

Founder of Living with Hearing Loss, Amy Morton, had a similar positive experience of opening up:

I was a beauty therapist and holistic organic therapist for twelve years. In that time I worked for a very busy salon in Leamington Spa and worked up to a senior level. During that time I was put on reception. Because I just 'got on with it' I struggled quietly at the start, worried that I would lose my job, and weakly voiced my view that I was struggling until one day I said firmly, 'I'm sorry, I can't work on reception. I'm finding it very difficult, so please don't assign me to the desk.' They were supportive, and I was assigned to doing what I do best!

Recently, I went on *Loose Women*. The team there were excellent at communicating in a way I felt comfortable with, and checking in with me about any needs I might have. I realise I'm in the privileged position of being an established actor and spokesperson, but hopefully these experiences will be commonplace for everyone in the industry in the future.

In fact, Sophie went on to say:

> More doors are opening and investment is being made into young, upcoming talent, especially with the celebration of sign language having artistic and inclusive value as opposed to being seen as the charity model of a communication tool reserved to 'help' those 'in need'. Being visible is now having a positive ripple effect on opportunities, education and achievements, which is a wave many deaf people are riding right now. Who knows how long we'll be able to ride it for, but the work must never stop.

This is awesome news!

I also worried about my job as a radio presenter, and whether my new hearing aid would affect my hire-ability. I mean, whoever has heard of a deaf radio presenter?! Thankfully, I can still present on the radio. I am clear about my communication needs for phone-ins (text-ins work really well), and I always ask to be able to see anyone I am interviewing or being interviewed by. I am even working with some radio stations behind the scenes to suggest more deaf-friendly processes. If you are ever asked to go on the radio, as long as you tell them in advance they should be able to sort a FaceTime scenario if you are being interviewed remotely. You can also ask to see the questions in advance. At times I get some negative comments on social media about being a deaf person on the radio, as it is not deaf friendly – but, as we have explored, deafness encompasses a range of different experiences and many deaf people and those with hearing loss do listen to the radio. I would rather work in an area I enjoy, ensure there is representation, and try and change things from the inside than avoid it altogether. I think that the radio and podcasts can be accessible, and it's all about raising awareness to make them more so.

My hearing aid really hasn't held me back: in fact, it's given me a new passion for activism and has opened up a whole new chapter of my career. My deafness is actually the reason I started writing books – and look where we are now! Some other deaf individuals have also found or created jobs that work well for them. For example, Lucy Rogers became an illustrator, using her heightened perception to record the world around her. Many deaf people become self-employed and have careers that involve working from home. As Lucy Rogers explains: 'I prefer it this way. I'm not sure how I would be able to cope in an office full of hearing people with no deaf awareness.' In fact, the Inklusion Guide, created for the publishing industry, states that 'over 600,000 disabled people in the UK are self-employed'.[69]

Being self-employed can give us the freedom to control our environment so it is accessible. It also means we can take time off when we need to for chronic conditions, concentration fatigue and to look after our mental health without trying to explain to an employer, who may challenge your reasons for wanting time off. Office environments can be particularly inaccessible for deaf people due to their layout, acoustics, lack of deaf awareness training, and also the daily commute to and from the office. My home office has become a safe haven compared to the audist environments I am often thrust into. It is worth noting that being self-employed is a privilege that some people can't take advantage of, due to lack of finances (for home office and job equipment) and support (learning business skills, negotiating fees, filing self-employed tax returns, knowing their self-employed rights, etc.).

Luke Christian, activist and owner of Deaf Identity, created his fashion brand to celebrate deafness: 'I wanted to mix my love of fashion with raising deaf awareness.' However, it has not been without its struggles. Luke told me: 'It's been a struggle to be taken seriously sometimes, and people often think I'm a charity. It's also been difficult to find help and support for disabled business owners too, but as the brand grows over time, I'm hoping things will change and people will start to take Deaf Identity seriously within the fashion and business world.' Despite his struggles, Luke's clothes have been featured in the press and worn by prominent deaf role models like Rose Ayling-Ellis, who wore a Deaf Identity T-shirt on *Strictly Come Dancing*. Luke also designed one of the T-shirts for Comic Relief 2022, which were sold across the UK.

The positives of being a deaf person at work

There are so many positives to being a deaf person in the workplace. Working with others and getting out of the house are both good for your mental health (when the workplace is accessible, that is). Work also gives you independence and a sense of accomplishment.

Keighley Miles talks about the joy of working in childcare as a deaf person:

> The children know once they get my attention they have my full attention. They don't have my full ears but they have my eyes, my body language, my facial expressions, and this teaches them that communication isn't just your mouth and ears; it's your whole body. They learn about people with different abilities from an early age.

She goes on:

> My deafness means I have to get creative about understanding stuff that relies on sound, and I use that creativity to design activities for the children, often on the spur of the moment.

Being deaf brings its own set of skills that hearing people haven't developed in the same way. Actor Nadia Nadarajah explains her heightened perception: 'I use my eyes a lot to look around and spot details. I observe so much with my ears switched off.' Having to lip-read and be aware of social cues has definitely made me a better communicator and interviewer. When I interview people on my podcast or on the radio, I always ask to be able to see the person – mainly to lip-read, but also so I can read subtle nuances in physicality and even breath patterns that tell me how they're feeling. I can tell whether someone I am interviewing is comfortable answering certain questions, whether I can push them further, when they are likely to stop speaking so I can ask my next question, and even when they are distracted and might need a wee break.

Nurse Asha explains how this skill comes in handy in life-or-death situations too: 'I am hyper-aware of people's body language, which comes naturally to me because I rely on lip-reading and body language to know what is going on, especially working in an ICU environment, where it's vital to get it right the first time in a sensitive situation.'

While being deaf brings its own positives to the workplace, we are also individuals with our own unique experiences and skills to share. Annie Harris says: 'I thrive in environments where employers see beyond my deafness and value the skills and knowledge I bring to the table.'

So, employers, why wouldn't you hire a deaf person?

Workplace tips

Amy Morton, founder of Living with Hearing Loss, says: 'I currently work online, so I always ensure I use a good platform to host video calls. My favourite is Google Meet – the captions are so much better than on other options.'

It can be useful to have a colleague who agrees to be a safe port of call for you, someone you feel comfortable around and who can make you feel less alone in challenging work scenarios. It is worth pointing out that this person is not a support worker. Support workers are trained to provide support and are paid for their time.

Jasper Williams says:

> I find it helpful to have a 'safe work buddy' too. This is someone who you can sit next to who has a bit more understanding and makes you feel safe/slightly less anxious

in work situations. Maybe you can signal to them, and they will come up with an excuse to go with you for a 1:1 lunch break instead of with everyone else. Put your needs first, as you will be most productive that way! And remember, if you really feel there needs to be more understanding, you can get your workplace Deaf awareness training through an Access to Work grant!

Chapter 13
Owning your deafness

'Hearing is something people take for granted, so for a person who is experiencing a hearing loss, it's a big shock,' explains illustrator Lucy Rogers. I couldn't agree more. My hearing loss was a *huge* shock: I'm talking 'jaw-on-the-floor, never-considered-it, thought-the-audiologist-was-joking' shock. However, as Blogger Bethan Harvey says, 'to me deafness is a normal part of life, as I've never known any different'. These might be very different beginnings to a deaf journey, but either way the individual will at some stage need to accept their deafness and deal with the way society responds to them because of it.

For author Jaipreet Virdi, her only identifier of deafness was how others responded, which she describes in her book *Hearing Happiness: Deafness Cures in History*: 'For a long time, I never understood that I lost my hearing. I believed the world had changed and everyone simply stopped noticing me'.[70]

Keighley Miles describes her experience: 'I had never met or heard of a deaf person. There wasn't the internet, like there is these days. I very quickly became worried about standing out and trying to hide that I spoke "funny".'

I can relate to this: the only deaf person I'd ever seen on TV was in the film *Four Weddings and a Funeral*, and that was a deaf person who used BSL, which I didn't. So often we see set ideas of deafness, such as someone who was born deaf and speaks with BSL, or Grandad who hasn't turned his hearing aids on so everyone is shouting during Christmas dinner. There is nothing wrong with these deaf experiences, but many people don't see themselves reflected in them – and that contributes to feelings of otherness. I remember leaving my audiologist's office with leaflets full of images of people with grey hair, dressed in cosy sweaters – they reminded me of an advert for dentures. (My gran wore dentures. I once walked into her bedroom and saw her teeth sitting in a glass on her bedside table and was scarred for life.) I didn't feel that I was being represented in those leaflets, and I remember feeling like the only person under eighty to ever need a hearing aid. If only I'd had model and entrepreneur Luke Christian with me at the time. He said: 'My advice for somebody who has discovered they are deaf or have hearing loss is to not panic or be sad.'

Luke, I am sorry to say I did both of those things.

When you are told you are deaf, you might react in a number of different ways. You might feel shocked, in denial, or angry. Amplifon audiologist Jane Noble agrees: 'Accepting hearing loss can be tricky! Some individuals may experience all the stages of grief and take some time to accept their hearing loss, while others may accept it for what it is and seek help immediately.' I definitely experienced a grief for my hearing, and there was crying in public places – and hiding out at home too.

As a teacher at a school for deaf children Victoria Sylvester explains how deafness affects the children she teaches:

Deafness doesn't just affect hearing; we support students with many things linked to their deafness, such as language development, and their emotional needs, such as coming to terms with their disability and feeling confident in talking about what they need. Also, many of our students struggle to understand how others are feeling, so we support them to learn about social situations.

If you are experiencing feelings of grief or you feel you need some support, please do reach out to someone. Close friends and relatives can be there for you, even though they might not have direct experience of what you are going through. There are also lots of organisations that do understand: you will find a list on p. 311. If you don't want to talk right now, the internet can be a great source of information and support (just make sure you are reading websites that are accredited sources). Lots of the charities mentioned in this book have helpful articles and lists of frequently asked questions on their websites, as well as profiles of awesome deaf people whose stories you may relate to. Searching 'deaf' on Instagram and TikTok can also lead to some great deaf content creators that you can follow and learn from. Please remember that you are not alone.

Advocating and activism

It took me some time to accept my hearing loss and deafness. I tried to ignore it for so long, but it was stand-up comedy that finally helped me begin to process my deafness through talking about it, and my experiences with it, on stage. I process life through talking, exploring and finding the funny in my hardest moments, and I found that opening up about it in a public arena meant that I began to draw others to me who were going through similar experiences. This joy in finding others who could relate led me to finding the Royal National Institute for Deaf People online and contacting them to say that I wanted to be involved in the work they were doing. Volunteering with RNID was a huge change for me: I started to own my deafness through working with other deaf people and campaigning for change and accessibility. Today I am proud to be an ambassador for RNID and to work with them on campaigns from the House of Commons to the cinema to make life easier for deaf people and people with hearing loss.

Another way of owning your deafness is to become an advocate for the community. Annie Harris, RNID advocacy officer, says: 'We live in a world where society is full of hearing privilege. It needs to change, and advocacy is how. We need to speak up and tell the world about us, to break through the barriers and seek meaningful social change.'

Doing this really helped me. Annie goes on: 'We want society to learn and understand the truth about the deaf community, so they can treat us with respect.'

Angela Barnes agrees: 'I think it's really important to talk about things. Even if you only have a small following on Twitter, I think it's important for people to hear.'

Whether speaking out about your experience is for you or not, as deaf people we all have to self-advocate – often so we can get what we need, whether this is better communication or better accessibility. This can be as simple as telling a friend that you'd like to find a quieter table at the back of the restaurant, to avoid background noise, or informing your workplace that you wear hearing aids. Charlotte Hyde says:

When you tell people that you're deaf, they will be looking to you to give them the answers. Don't panic. You won't know what works for you right off the bat. Explain that you're learning yourself and you want to take some time to experiment. Tell them that if you need them to do anything differently, you'll let them know.

Self-advocacy can simply mean standing up for yourself and having confidence in who you are. However, it can be difficult to stay confident in the face of negative or frustrating reactions. BSL tutor Fletch@ explains:

I feel that if I respond [during a conversation], [the hearing person] will continue to talk and turn their face away, not realising that I can't see/understand what they are saying. If I respond by letting them know I am deaf, I always feel that they are either patronising and take pity on me or avoid trying to communicate. But there's nothing wrong with me! Don't allow people to make you feel bad for being deaf.

I was asked on social media how to self-advocate as a deaf person. It's quite a hard question to answer. I think my first response would be: take your time. No one is expecting you to get a hearing aid and then a week later be educating others or giving speeches on the importance of deaf awareness. I'm only six years into my deaf journey, and I'm still learning so much all the time. I have also learned a lot from the people I interviewed for this book. Doing research and listening to others in the community can definitely inform your own advocacy, as Charlotte Hyde agrees: 'If I hadn't enrolled on that BSL module at uni, I wouldn't be who I am today. Learning about my community, my history and my language honestly changed my entire perception of my deafness and my sense of self. I have to credit Ilan Dwek, my amazing tutor, who completely changed my life.'

Learning is so important, but at some point there are certain things you need to decide for yourself. You need to stay true to what feels right for you. For some this process will happen naturally. As a performer, I wanted to immerse myself in this new deaf world and discover more about it and talk about the process on stage. I don't know everything there is to know about being deaf – who does? – but I'm happy to talk about my process and my learning so far. I'm also happy to be proven wrong by a more informed person. I will, however, always stand up for my beliefs, even when others may disagree, because I have always been 'an outspoken little madam', as a babysitter once called me. On the other hand, if you have not always been 'an outspoken little madam' like me, this process might take a little longer for you. Charlotte Hyde says: 'Self-advocacy is hard and takes tremendous courage, but in time it will become easier. There will also be days where you don't have the energy to self-advocate or "stand out" as different. This is completely okay, and it absolutely isn't a failure on your part.'

Pride

It may sound odd to you that people are proud of being deaf, but we are. Hopefully by this point you will understand a little of why, but straight after being told you have hearing loss, you might struggle to see a day when you'll be proud, or even happy, about being part of the deaf community. Actor Sophie Stone explains: 'It's taken me a long time to come to this point:

to shed the internal audism by external attitudes and negative language that surrounds it.'

I can relate as I realised I had to overcome my own built-in opinions of what being deaf meant and how that looks. These internal opinions develop over time, often during our childhood, by hearing and seeing certain attitudes towards, or depictions of, deaf people. I had to work hard to overcome my own inherent prejudices towards deaf and disabled people before I could come to terms with the fact that I was now both of those things. It's a process, like breaking up with a partner, of healing and being ready to love again.

BSL tutor Fletch@ says: 'I would advise people to be proud of being deaf as there is nothing wrong with it. Be happy with who you are, and if other people cannot accept it or are not happy to try to adapt, that is their problem, not yours.' I totally agree. Often acceptance comes with a new-found pride, and it is a wonderful feeling.

Pride comes from honouring your own experience as well as that of those who have gone before you. Knowing a little deaf history can also inform your deaf pride.

*

The London Asylum for the Deaf and Dumb on the Old Kent Road in London was founded in 1792. Deaf people were sent to live here by their families. While descriptions of the institution suggest it was a place of education to 'save' deaf children, imagine your loved ones packing you off to live in an asylum! The Oxford Dictionary defines asylum as 'a hospital where people who were mentally ill could be cared for, often for a long time'. But these people were deaf, not mentally ill! Another relevant moment in history was when thirty-one centres were set up around the UK after the First World War to help rehabilitate and support the 30,000 soldiers 'deafened in the war'.[71] I had no idea about this until I began researching for this book. It's a result of the war that doesn't seem to be covered in documentaries or history books. Soldiers becoming deaf in war still happens today, and there is an Armed Forces Compensation Scheme[72] for soldiers who have been affected. Any soldier who has hearing loss from serving after 2005 can apply. That brings us up to BSL becoming legally recognised as a language in 2022. In between these events there is a wealth of deaf history that is worth researching to help you feel pride in your own deafness, when you see how far we have come.

Finding your community is so important, not only for your mental health but also for owning your deafness. I have learned so much about myself – and deafness as a whole – by meeting other deaf people, reading their work and following them on social media. As actor Sophie Stone advises:

Don't try to beat the culture, join it. Get wiser, bolder and own exactly who you are. Learn BSL, respect it and yourself, and stop apologising for existing. Instead of 'I can't hear', choose 'I don't hear'. Instead of 'Sorry, I'm deaf,' choose 'I'm deaf' – and see what adjustments are made. Don't waste energy or pain on those who don't value who you are, what you need, or what you've been through. Unpack the audism you've been conditioned to believe, then own your space.

Charlotte Hyde, deaf activist, reveals:

To me, my deafness is probably the best bit about myself. I truly love being deaf. That feeling of taking your hearing aids off at the end of a long day? Bliss. Being able to switch off when the world gets too noisy? Incredible. Tangible benefits to deafness aside, I believe I wouldn't be the same person I am today if I wasn't deaf. Being deaf defines me in the best way. It has made me a more compassionate person, taught me the importance of clear communication, and has gifted me with a community, culture, and language that I love.

Chapter 14
Travelling with hearing loss

'If you're deaf or have hearing loss, service providers have a duty to make reasonable adjustments so you are able to access their services. Failure to do so could be unlawful discrimination,' says RNID.

This includes public transport.

Public transport

Public transport was one of the biggest bugbears of the deaf people I interviewed. I'm a non-driver, so public transport is how I get around most of the time. While I'm grateful it exists and appreciate its connections, especially in London, I too get so frustrated by the lack of accessibility. Keighley Miles reveals:

> When I started to travel by myself, I struggled. It would be things such as a change of direction on the bus or a train was no longer stopping at a station because of XYZ, and I would never hear the announcement and often ended up in a place I wasn't meant to be. I had no confidence getting public transport because I was scared, so I ended up never going out.

Travelling can be nerve-racking for people who are deaf. A lack of accessibility means that many people simply don't put themselves through it; instead, they stay at home, becoming isolated, which is damaging to their mental health. BSL tutor Fletch@ explains: 'All of my life, I have hated public transport because I can't hear what's going on or what people are saying.'

This doesn't just mean announcements; it might be staff at train ticket barriers/platforms, bus drivers shouting inform-ation from the front of the bus, ticket conductors, etc. It doesn't help that train stations are not acoustically pleasant, often with high ceilings that bounce the noise around, no soft furnishings, and people speaking through Perspex screens. You can imagine how much more difficult this was when everyone was wearing masks too! Even the insides of trains and buses are not sound insulated, so you can hear the sounds of the wheels on the tracks or on the road and other outside noises as well as noises inside the carriage. For those who struggle with background noise, public transport environments can be overwhelming. In 2017 I was involved with a TV programme called *Upfront* on BBC One, which investigated rising sound levels in London. While I went to bars in Soho to measure the decibel levels (and, yes, have a cocktail or two), a journalist sat on each Tube line in Zones 1 and 2 to measuring the decibel level. (Yes, I realise I got the easy job there.) London's Northern Line and Central Line came off worst, with noises rising to a damaging level. I spoke to Dr Joe Sollini of University College London's Ear Institute for the programme, and he said the study was 'concerning'. I would go so far to say that it is outrageous. We know that repeated exposure to noise above 85 dB can damage your hearing. Levels over 95 dB were recorded on the Tube. These levels were not for prolonged periods of time during one journey, but if you made that journey every day to and from work or worked in that environment (e.g. train drivers), this would be a potentially damaging exposure that could affect your hearing over the long term. In fact, in 2019 Transport for London agreed to provide over-the-ear ear defenders for staff who requested them, thanks to a campaign run by the train drivers' union ASLEF, which was unsatisfied with the ear plugs provided.[73]

I think more needs to be done to address the potentially damaging sound levels on public transport for deaf and hearing people alike. This study was carried out in London, but I would welcome a study of public transport (tubes, metros, trams, trains and buses) across the UK to monitor sound levels. Sound insulation and acoustic panels could be used, as well as compulsory ear defenders for staff, then new plans should be drawn up to design new train carriages, for example, which take sound into consideration at the initial building stages.

I would love to change the public transport network to be more sound aware and more accessible for deaf people, but what can deaf people do in the meantime? Amy Morton says: 'When travelling, I make a plan ahead of my journey and speak to someone, if I can, to get updates, as I can't always hear the voiceover announcements. I make sure I know how many stops it is to my stop.' Similarly, illustrator Lucy Rogers explains: 'I'm constantly checking my phone for train updates on time changes or delays, etc., because I can't rely on hearing what the voice overhead is saying. I quite often have to follow other people if I notice everyone leaving the platform, but I have no idea what is going on.' While there are screens on platforms, often they do not announce platform changes or announcements. Apps can be useful for accessing transport, so downloading a local travel app, bus app or the National Rail app should give you real-time information when you travel. Lucy says: 'Trains really need to improve their system and provide more subtitles somewhere for any broadcastings.' Quite often, the screens on trains are broken or not switched on, and announcements at large stations are audio only with no subtitling, even though many screens are available. The frustrating thing is that you can have everything in place, such as apps on your phone giving you information on your journey, but things can still go wrong. Luke Christian explains: 'I've had a few incidents where the train has ground to a halt and we've been held up. Almost every time, I've never been able to understand what is going on due to the train driver announcing updates through speakers, while there are no screens.' Fletch@ reveals a similar experience: 'I was with an interpreter getting on the train. I checked the Trainline app to confirm the platform. On the way there, my interpreter told me there had been an announcement advising everybody there was a change of platform. I checked the Trainline app again and the platform had not changed! We rushed to reach the platform and ended up missing the train.' Travelling with a hearing companion, while not always possible, is useful to help navigate this. And as a deaf person you can apply for a Disabled Persons Railcard, which gives you and a companion one-third off your tickets (see the section on p. 222 for how to apply).

And there is hope that this may change in future. Audiologist Adam Chell says: 'In the future, with the advancement of Bluetooth capabilities, hearing aids will be able to connect to tannoy systems in train stations [so deaf people] can hear the announcements crystal clear.' While many train stations have hearing loop facilities, they are often broken or not switched on, but that's worth a try until the Bluetooth capability is introduced.

Buses and trams often have screens displaying the names of stops; however, these may also be switched off or broken, and they are no use if the bus is diverted to a different route. Even if the screens are working, I use a bus app and a maps app on my phone to track buses in real time so I know where I am and can work out where I need to get off. But it's not possible to prepare for everything. Fletch@ remembers:

> One time I was sitting at the back of a bus, the bus pulled over (not in a regular bus stop). Everybody was talking, the driver got out, came back on and said something . . . People came down from the top and got off, as well as people around me. I sat on my own at the back of the bus, wondering what was going on. It turned out there was smoke and fire coming from the outside of the back of the bus, close to where I was sitting. I felt so confused and anxious.

Of course, in this case the driver should have done a full evacuation, rather than making an announcement, but when something unexpected happens in real life, things aren't always done by the book.

While we can use apps, bring a hearing companion, and use hearing loops, nothing replaces old-fashioned human kindness. If you see a person sitting at the back of the bus while everyone else is evacuating it, please show common sense and kindness and help them. Motioning for that person to come with you then explaining clearly what was happening when they are off the bus (type it out on your phone if lip-reading isn't working) would have been the thing to do. Learning 'can I help?' Or 'are you okay?' in sign language would take two minutes and could really help in a situation like this.

Getting a Disabled Persons Railcard

A Disabled Persons Railcard gives you and a companion one-third off rail travel. You can apply for one online at www.disabledpersons-railcard.co.uk. If you have hearing loss or are D/deaf, you are eligible for the railcard. The website states:

You are eligible for the Disabled Persons Railcard if you:

- receive Personal Independence Payment or Adult Disability Payment (ADP)
- receive Disability Living Allowance or Child Disability Payment at either:
  - the higher or lower rate for the mobility component, or
  - the higher or middle rate for the care component
- have a visual impairment
- have a hearing impairment
- have epilepsy
- receive Attendance Allowance, Severe Disablement Allowance or Pension Age Disability Payment (PADP)
- receive War Pensioner's Mobility Supplement
- receive War or Service Disablement Pension for 80 per cent or more disability
- buy or lease a vehicle through the Motability scheme[74]

Yes, I know that 'hearing impairment' is outdated language. I contacted the organisation via social media and email and asked them nicely to change it. Let's see if they listen.

The website explains how to apply for the railcard. You will need to submit proof of your deafness: I applied by uploading copies of my hearing tests, which I got from my audiologist. The railcard costs £20 for a year or £54 for three years. It does not give you a discount on Eurostar.

Driving

Yes, deaf people can drive. I can't drive, so I am a bad advocate for this, but that's mainly because I like to be driven around by my loved ones, pretending they are my chauffeurs while I lounge around in the back of a limo (aka Ford Focus).

Keighley Miles says: 'As soon as I could, I learned to drive just so I didn't have to use public transport or even taxis.' Blogger Bethan Harvey explains: 'Deaf people, believe it or not, can drive. I am one of those who can. Deaf people are much more visual, and so they can rely on using their mirrors (more hearing people need to do this) to see, e.g. if an emergency vehicle is coming. Although it cannot always be heard, the flashing lights can be seen, and you can observe other cars and vehicles moving out of the way.'

In fact, a study has shown that deaf people are actually better drivers than hearing people: 'Deaf people make better drivers than people with normal hearing – and they could be the world's safest motorists, a fascinating new study shows . . . That's because they compensate for their disability by concentrating on watching the road.'[75]

Just another reason to be proud to be deaf!

You don't have to tell the DVLA you are deaf if you have a car or motorcycle licence. If you have a bus, coach or lorry licence, however, you must tell the DVLA that you are deaf.

Travelling abroad

Will my hearing-aid batteries explode during take-off? Can I wear my hearing aids when going through a metal detector? These were two of the exciting questions I had when I travelled abroad on an aeroplane for the first time since discovering I was deaf. Just to ease your mind, no, your hearing-aid batteries (or your hearing aids, or your ears) generally won't explode during take-off. Phew. Also, you don't have to take your hearing aids out to go through the metal detector – or point them out to staff. I've also travelled with hearing-aid batteries in my hand luggage, and this has been fine.

Your hearing aids can actually help you on a flight, as audiologist Adam Chell explains: 'A lot of hearing aids have a nice mute feature for noisy aeroplanes or trains. They then act like a fancy pair of earplugs. You can also stream music or films directly to your hearing aids from your phone or computer.' No more ill-fitting plane headphones that are handed out with the hospital blue blankets! It is important to remember, though, that if you're on a long flight and want to watch/listen to the online entertainment system, you will need to bring your own over-the-ear headphones to plug into the monitor, as the inflight team usually only provides in-ear ones.

Blogger Bethan Harvey reveals: 'I love travelling abroad, but I don't do well with take-off and landing. It absolutely terrifies me. I hate the pressure of it and the thought of my left ear popping (my right physically cannot). When it has popped on take-off or landing I literally cannot hear anything at all, and it takes some time for it to pop again.' Tinnitus UK has some advice for travelling comfortably:

- Sit in the front of the plane where the engine noise isn't as loud. Anywhere in front of the wings will be an advantage.
- Swallow and yawn as much as possible. This will open the Eustachian tube and allow air to enter the middle ear. When outside air pressure changes, the Eustachian tube supplies a bubble of air and the ears pop. When this happens, air pressure has been equalised.
- Chew gum or suck on a sweet. It will cause you to swallow more often and help equalise the air pressure during take-off and descent.
- Stay awake during descent. The descent is the part of the plane ride where you will have a harder time adjusting to the pressure changes. Your Eustachian tube and ears don't adjust as well when you are sleeping, so it's important to stay awake.
- Try to avoid flying if you have a cold or upper respiratory infection, as it can make it more difficult for your Eustachian tube to operate.
- A nasal decongestant may be helpful. Even if you are not suffering from a cold, this may help keep those airways and tubes open for better pressure release.
- Leave your hearing aids in place, as you may find them particularly helpful during a flight.[76]

When you are travelling, you may need to interact with some people who haven't had deaf awareness training, so unfortunately you will need to pack your patience along with your Hawaiian shirt and sun cream. Co-founder and co-artistic director at Hot Coals Productions, Clare-Louise English, says:

'We once asked at the airport if we could make sure I sat with my friend on the plane so that she could interpret if I needed it. The person replied that, as I was disabled, she'd put me in a window seat! I guess that was so I could see where we were going!?' Living with Hearing Loss founder Amy Morton shares: 'If cabin crew are wearing masks on a plane, I always make sure a cabin crew member knows I have hearing loss for safety reasons: if they are asking me or telling me something in an emergency, it's important that they know I'm not going to understand unless they lower their mask.'

I agree: it's useful to let cabin crew know you are deaf for health and safety reasons. It also means that you can request better seats and you can be seated next to your companion without incurring an extra charge.

Chapter 15

Deaf dating and having sex

Trigger warning for this chapter: abuse and sexual assault.

Ooh, this chapter feels risqué, doesn't it?! Deafness and sex – what a taboo. When I spoke to other deaf people, sex and dating while deaf came up again and again. It's something we don't really talk about. You will be pleased to hear that deaf people have sex, though, and it's just as great as hearing people's sex, if not better (because we pay less attention to the couple arguing next door). There are a few things to be aware of if you are having sex with a deaf person, and I will delve into these below (yes, I know 'delve' is an excellent word to use in a chapter about sex. You're welcome).

Dating

In 2022, ITV reality dating show *Love Island* had its first deaf contestant, Tasha Ghouri, who has a cochlear implant. This was the first time I had seen a young deaf person represented in the modern dating world, and at first it felt positive and inclusive. However, Tasha received a lot of backlash online and via social media, with people mocking her voice and even saying they wanted to 'rip out her implant'. I found these ableist threats seriously worrying, especially at a time when deaf people are proudly talking about their deaf experiences and even including the fact that they're deaf on their online dating profiles. Would the public reaction to Tasha have a negative impact on deaf people dating in the real world? Tasha didn't have a smooth ride on the show, but she ended up meeting someone and finding love. In her final speech on the show to her partner Andrew Le Page, she said: 'The fact that when I fall asleep and you take out the cochlear implant for me – that's how I know you're the one.' My ex-husband never took my hearing aid out for me – perhaps that's why our relationship didn't work!

Tasha calls her deafness her 'superpower', a word that does not resonate with many in the deaf community; it's usually used by hearing people trying to reframe deafness. I encourage you to use, and identify with, whichever terms work for you, but finding out the history of such terms can also be useful.

Tasha was open about her cochlear implant from the beginning of the show and found love, so if you're worried that your deafness might affect someone's feelings towards you, you can see Tasha's experience as a positive example. But how will your deafness impact the experience?

When I was dating after my divorce, there were a lot of new factors I had to get used to. When introducing myself, I had some new descriptors to add. First of all, I was divorced, and even if I had wanted to hide this information, I have a podcast about the subject (The Divorce Social – check it out!), so I couldn't really escape talking about it when people asked me what I did. I came out as bisexual after my divorce, and navigating that, particularly on queer dating apps, where some gay women unmatched me because I wasn't 'fully gay', was a new experience. I'm also deaf, wear a hearing aid, and lip-read. So when should you tell people these facts about yourself? In your dating app profile? For example: 'I like knitting, reading, having sex with all genders, taking my hearing aid out after a long day, and Nando's. PS I am also divorced.'

Or do you work it into the first conversation you have online?

ME: Would you rather have a rabbit's tail or a squirrel's tail growing from your bottom?

THEM: Ha ha, erm . . . rabbit's, I guess, as I could hide it in my trousers.

ME: Would you rather your date be divorced, deaf or bisexual? Or all three?

THEM: . . .

I know – I'm fun to chat with online. Or you could wait until you meet your date then eke out the information. Or wait until things get serious . . . but then you'd be in the bedroom saying, 'You pop off your socks and I will pop out my hearing aid.' No, that's probably too late. Dancer Sarah Adedeji says: 'You just don't know how the person will respond to that information being disclosed, and it can make or break a relationship that's already starting to build.'

So, when do you tell someone you are deaf? Activist Charlotte Hyde reveals:

I used to wait to tell people I met on dating apps face to face, but honestly, being upfront and putting 'I'm deaf' in my bio significantly increased the quality of the matches I got. Personally, I avoided anyone who asked me to teach them BSL, or who made a big deal out of the way my voice might sound before they met me. If the person I matched with asked me about being deaf, then I'd just tell them how I communicate and ask if they had any questions.

There's much better advice here from Charlotte than from me, I think!

Worrying about being judged for who you are is part of dating, whether or not you have a disability, although we may worry a little more than most hearing people. However, as Charlotte Hyde says: 'No date I've had so far has had an issue with it, which is something I wish I could tell my teenage self.' It's important to remember that your date will be worrying much more about themselves than about you: they will have their own insecurities and will hope that you will accept them for who they are. Being kind is always a good idea on a date – and hopefully you will get kindness back.

Once you've found someone you'd like to date, you need to decide where to meet them. This can be a minefield, as date venues can stop a good date turning into a great date. Often I used to let my dates choose where to meet, but then I'd arrive at a tiny, dark, very loud bar where hearing my date, or even lip-reading, was virtually impossible. I think finding your ideal dating spot and sticking to it works well – at least you know the venue will be a good match! You might like to use the SoundPrint app to find some quiet bars in your area (see p. 131). Actor Nadia Nadarajah told me that she suggests dinner or bowling for a date activity that provides easier communication. She explained: 'With hearing people I've always got to make sure I have pen and paper with me so it's ready if needed. When I meet them and see how they communicate – if they're easy to lip-read, then great, we can communicate that way, taking our time, adding in some gestures to make sure we're understood. Sometimes there's a bit of grin-and-bear-it.'

I actually ended up speaking about my 'dating while deaf' experiences on the radio to raise awareness. After meeting presenter Jeremy Vine at a book launch and regaling him with my tales, I was invited on to his BBC Radio 2 show to talk about my tips for dating while deaf. Interestingly, while I talked about dates I had been on, I didn't mention whether I was single or in a relationship during the radio segment, and afterwards on social media I had three date offers from listeners! So there you go: there are lots of people who will date you if you are deaf. Just go on the radio to talk about it. While radio isn't always accessible for deaf people, the brilliant people at RNID did create a transcript for my interview so that everyone could enjoy it. It is, of course, possible to find love as a deaf person – and your new partner doesn't need to be someone in the deaf community. Sarah Adedeji explains: 'I'm in a relationship with a hearing person who had never met a Deaf person before myself, and they've pretty much taken it in their stride and are learning something new every day, happily.'

So, what are my top tips for dating when deaf?

- Be open about your deafness. It might be scary at first, but it's better if your date is aware, so you can focus on fun date stuff. You can put it in your bio or let your date know before you meet.
- If you lip-read, let your date know that you will need to sit opposite them, rather than next to them, and you will need a venue with good lighting.

- You pick the venue, then you know you will be comfortable.
- Bring a hearing-aid charger/batteries if you think you might stay at your date's house overnight.
- Be kind.
- Have fun.

Tips for dating a deaf person

- Be led by your date on terminology, and whether they're happy talking about their deafness on the date. They might prefer to focus on other things.
- Pick an acoustically pleasant venue, or let them choose where you go.
- Ask if there is anything that would make the meet easier for them, like good lighting or you learning a little BSL.
- Don't make the 'what?' joke. Don't ask them to teach you BSL.
- Do some research: educate yourself about the deaf spectrum and Deaf history (this doesn't mean you need to bring up the subject on the date to show you've done it, though).
- Be kind.
- Have fun.

Sex while wearing hearing aids

So what is sex like with hearing aids? Or without hearing aids? Well, most audiologists don't tend to answer questions about sex; I asked them about wearing hearing aids at the gym instead to get the information I needed. I figured that sex is like a workout: sweaty, takes balance – and sometimes strength, and can be done in different locations. I have always taken my hearing aid out for the gym, which creates its own problems. Due to my one-sided hearing loss, my balance is affected. When I'm at the gym lifting weights, I'm more off-balance so I can fall over. Audiologist Adam Chell reveals: 'A lot of modern hearing aids have very good dust and water resistance. In fact, one manufacturer has just launched a completely waterproof hearing aid. I wouldn't recommend swimming in them, though; it just means that they are life-proof and very forgiving.' At least your partner can now lick your ear without fear of ruining your hearing aids! Amplifon audiologist Jane Noble advises: 'Take care to clean and inspect your hearing aids after your workout, and wipe off any moisture which has built up.' Presumably the same advice applies after sex . . .

The big question when it comes to sex is: hearing aids on or off? It's like socks. My advice there is, always take your socks off – but is it the same for hearing aids? Illustrator Lucy Rogers can't decide: 'I like having my hearing aids on sometimes and off sometimes, but I prefer to have them on in case I make too much noise for my neighbours.'

I can honestly say I don't think I have ever left my hearing aid on for sex in the bedroom – perhaps being a performer means I don't worry about being a noisy neighbour. Let them enjoy the performance! I followed Jane Noble's advice: 'Remember to take your hearing aids out if you're going for a swim or showering after exercise, and store them in a safe place while they're not in your ears.' Hearing aids mostly don't like water (unless they're snazzy waterproof ones), and when it comes to sex there's a lot of potential for liquids, so I have always taken mine out to be safe. That means no sexy shower scenes with your hearing aid in! Jane's last piece of advice, about storing your hearing aids in a safe place, is also very important. I once left my hearing aid, along with my earrings, on the bedside table of a sexual conquest (that wasn't his actual name). When I sneaked out in the early hours it took me a good hour to realise what I had left behind. I had to message him, apologising for sneaking out and asking if he could return my hearing aid the next morning. He returned it to a members' club in central London for me, in a brown envelope, which made it all feel much more serious, like I was getting a letter from HMRC or something. It was actually a good life lesson in always being nice to people you sleep with; I have never sneaked out on someone again.

So we know I take mine out – but what's it like if you leave your hearing aids in? Charlotte Hyde says: 'The best way I can describe it is like static. Especially if you're near any fabrics that can rub against the microphones on your hearing aids.' Clare-Louise English describes the experience as:

> So much worry! What if they put their hand on my ear and my hearing aid squeaks? What if they run their hand through my hair and feel my hearing aid? Should I take my hearing aid out now? If I leave it in, will it squeak? When would be a good time to take it out so they don't notice? What if it's dark? I won't be able to lip-read or hear. What if I fall asleep with my hearing aid in? What if they see it on my bedside? Is now a good time to tell them I'm deaf so I can stop worrying about all of the above? Afterwards, shall I say, 'I'm taking my hearing aid out now so I can go to sleep, but I won't be able to hear you starting from now?'

So it's not just practicalities that can be worrying; some deaf people worry about their partner seeing their hearing aid. Feeling an unexpected lump on someone's head could take you out of the sexy moment if you weren't expecting it, and no matter how honest I have been with my dates, they always stare a bit the first time I take out my hearing aid. Perhaps the answer here is to make sure they know about your hearing aid before you hit the bedroom (I understand this is not always possible) and perhaps you could even show it to them beforehand so they can look at it and get all their curiosity out before things get more intimate. When I began to write this section of the book, I realised I had never let my current partner have a good look at my hearing aid, despite being very open about it and telling them how it works and my accessibility needs.

But what if you don't wear hearing aids? How is your sex life affected? Actor Nadia Nadarajah explains: 'Well, of course, we use light [for lip-reading and BSL], so need that switched on, or can turn a lamp on. Without light, we'd be in the dark – in more ways than one. If my partner is deaf, or a hearing person that knows sign, then we can do deafblind manual fingerspelling on the palm and touch in the dark to communicate.' I'd like to try fingerspelling in this environment – it sounds like it could be particularly sensual, if you were in the mood.

Sex positions

What is a deaf person's favourite sex position? Whatever feels the nicest. When it comes to sex positions, there are also some things to consider: comfort, flexibility, the amount of effort you want to put in, and whether your partner is deaf. If you are new to having sex and you're thinking, 'Oh God, there's something else to learn', don't worry. It all gets easier – and usually lazier – over time. For example, doggy-style (where one of you is on all fours, like a dog, and the other stands or kneels behind you) can be great, but not if you want to have a chat during sex, as it's not a very lip-reading-friendly position unless you are having sex with an owl (which you shouldn't. I'm sure it's illegal). Any position where you are facing away from your partner can be difficult for communication, as can having sex in the dark, as Nadia mentioned earlier. A lot of the time you need to weigh up the merits of harsh, possibly unflattering, lighting so you can lip-read versus a ban on oral communication. Charlotte Hyde explains: 'Whispering just isn't a thing in my bedroom, and the lights have to be left on. Sex is typically associated with more hushed tones, but I can't hear those. It isn't very sexy when you have to ask your partner to repeat themselves every time they say something!'

I can totally relate to this. During my time in stand-up comedy I spoke to a lot of women who liked their other halves to do some dirty talking in the bedroom, but a lot of straight men I spoke to found talking dirty embarrassing. So if you're in a straight relationship and you're trying to encourage your male partner to talk dirty, they will usually start out tentatively with some whispered sexy words. The issue is, while you want to praise them for coming out of their shell, you might have no idea what they're saying – and shouting 'Speak up! I can't hear your dirty talk!' doesn't exactly add to the mood. To avoid this, you might assume they are talking dirty to you and reply in the same vein, only to realise they were actually telling you they had to stop because they had cramp in their thigh. It can be a risky business to navigate.

The LGBTQIA+ community

As a bisexual woman, queer representation in the deaf community is important to me. And, yes, queer deaf people do exist!

Deaf Rainbow UK[77] provides information and resources for Deaf LGBTIQA+ people. These include an LGBT+ BSL glossary (I learned the sign for 'bisexual' on this site), coming-out stories, and information about where to seek help if you're suffering abuse in an LGBTQIA+ relationship.

Fetishes

There are some interesting fetishes out there. Your deafness, disability or hearing aid could be a fetish for someone who is not disabled. While many people see this as fetishised able-ism and wrong, some disabled people are happy to go along with it, as long as it's consensual. Emily Yates presented a BBC documentary investigating this world. She told the BBC News:

> I found myself being introduced to a community of people who are sexually aroused, and attracted to, disability, as friends pointed me towards some websites about people known as devotees. The websites would become the doorway to discovering some pretty dark stuff but, surprisingly, I found it strangely refreshing at times.[78]

When asked what the weirdest thing he had ever been told or asked by a non-disabled person, Deaf Identity founder Luke Christiansen tweeted that he was asked: 'Can I fuck you without your hearing aids in so you have no idea what I'll be saying or doing?' In my opinion this is fetishised ableism – someone getting off on the fact that you can't hear them, so they can do whatever they want. This rings 'sexual assault' alarm bells for me. As Emily Yates goes on to say in her interview: 'I think there's also a problem when you fetishise something, that it can hamper you from having feelings for the full person.' Letting someone do whatever they want to your body and mind requires constant consent and trust, and I don't think that's what's being expressed here. If you ever feel uncomfortable in a sexual environment, whether is it to do with your disability or not, you can stop. You don't have to do anything you don't want to do. You deserve respect, as does your disability, and constant consent is essential in all sexual encounters.

Chapter 16

Being deaf and your mental health

Trigger warning for this chapter: suicide and mental health conditions.

Sorry. Declining mental health is not exactly a fun topic, is it? But it's a necessary one to discuss. I don't bring it up to scare you. I think it's useful to know the stats around mental health for deaf people. It's a statistic we don't hear about very often, but it's important to talk about it.

Deaf Unity (https://deafunity.org/) is a charity whose mission is 'empowering deaf people by providing the right support at critical moments from youth to adulthood'. Its website states that 'Mental health issues affect 1 in 4 people in the UK every year, with worries about things like money, employment and health making it harder for people to cope. In the deaf community, worryingly this number rises to 1 in every 2.5 people (around 40 per cent) experiencing mental health issues.'

Audiologist Adam Chell says:

> Hearing loss can have a significant impact on mental health . . . the immediate impacts can include social isolation, loneliness, frustration, helplessness and despair. You then have long-term impacts such as cognitive decline, depression and social anxiety. And because of the feeling of shame,

embarrassment and often grief which people may feel, people would rather tolerate this than wear a hearing aid.

Audiologist Rita Kairouz, founder of Little Auricles, agrees: 'There are mental and emotional effects to hearing loss. They can include anxiety, depression, isolation, denial and anger. Unfortunately, social isolation and depression are common in deaf and hard-of-hearing people, and that's why changing the stigma is very important.'

At some point in my deaf journey I have felt all of these things. While there are so many positives to being deaf, the barriers put in our way by society can lead to depression, anxiety, and days when leaving the house and facing it all feels like too much to handle. Being in difficult situations because of my deafness can exacerbate my anxiety.

Sound is very emotive, and can be linked to our memory. There are sounds that immediately take us back to certain times in our lives. The song 'Glamorous' by Fergie will for ever transport me back to sitting in the back of a car driving through South Africa, playing third wheel to my friend who had just met her future husband. Turns out I'm a pretty great third wheel, as it all worked out for them. Luckily I can still enjoy music, even if I can't always hear the lyrics, but other sounds have been completely lost to me.

The disappearance or reappearance of sounds can be over-whelming. When I heard birdsong for the first time after I got my hearing aids, I was very emotional. I hadn't realised that I had been missing it for so long, but standing in my garden and hearing the blue tits singing brought me to tears. Founder of Living with Hearing Loss, Amy Morton, had a

240

similar experience with birdsong – in fact, she measured her hearing using it: 'From four years till when I was in my twenties I could hear a pigeon, but from my twenties, with improvements in technology, I was hearing higher-pitched birds like blue tits. Now, with my latest powerful aids, I can hear the most beautiful birdsong in my garden, which I am forever grateful for.' Comedian Angela Barnes says, 'I forgot that light switches made a sound when you clicked them.' Sometimes these seemingly small moments can have a huge impact.

Feeling excluded in a hearing world also has an impact. Keighley Miles explains: 'Being socially awkward/different had, and still has, a major effect on me. I'm still on medication for this. Even though I have accepted it and I'm proud to be deaf, it doesn't make the last thirty years of feeling like I didn't fit in any easier, or my feelings at that time any different.' Growing up knowing you're 'different' from other children can be tough, as can others' reactions to what makes you 'different'. Actor Sophie Stone describes the effect of these poor reactions:

People shouted at me for not listening and I was always told 'I couldn't': couldn't play, couldn't be a part of things, couldn't hear things, couldn't pass tests, couldn't say words properly. The number of 'couldn'ts' and 'can'ts' that were thrown at me, I started to believe them. Family gatherings and group dinners were the hardest. I realise now that I was always worried, but it was such a normal state of being that I stopped noticing how much it was affecting my relationships, my social behaviours, my growth. I didn't have language until I was seven, so that in itself shows the deprivation and mental health impact it had on me – not the deafness, but the lack of support and access I so desperately needed. If there was

241

positive framing and transparent support from the start, I would have had a very different start in life.

Blogger Bethan Harvey had a very difficult time during her teenage years:

> I received death threats on a regular basis, such as being told to go home and kill myself, if I didn't they'd do it for me, and vividly describing how. I was told I should kill myself, I deserved to die, everyone would be happier if I was dead. Regularly told [that] students would bring a gun or knife into school and kill me if I was too chicken to do it. I was threatened to be thrown overboard a ferry on a school trip, to name a few. This led to all sorts of issues growing up. It knocked and destroyed my confidence, self-belief and self-esteem ... I developed anger issues because I just didn't know how to deal with everything, and it led to me attempting to take my own life when I was in Year 9.

Looking back now, Bethan says:

> At one point or another we have all needed support, and there is no shame in it. Your support network of friends and family will often be the ones to get you through. Ensure that any medical teams and professionals are supportive and listen to you. If they're not, don't be afraid to ask for a second opinion or to switch professionals leading your care.

BSL tutor Fletch@ reveals: 'There have been times when I have felt so depressed, I have considered taking my own life. Twice.' While it was Bethan's support network that got her through these dark times, Fletch@ found solace in a new skill:

'SignSong really helped me get through times when I suffered with my mental health.'

Access to mental health services is a huge issue for the deaf community. A telephone service for booking GP appointments, nurses calling your name for your appointment, no BSL interpreters or speech-to-text services are all barriers to the deaf community who are seeking help. There are, however, mental health and deaf charities that offer accessible support options. For example, the Samaritans offer support via email and an app, and Mind extend that to post and an online chat function. Deaf Unity and Sign Health offer help with mental health services too. Mark Atkinson advises: 'Make the most of the support available. There's lots of information on our website to get you started (rnid.org.uk), or you can have a chat with someone at our contact centre over the phone or by email.'

How change can impact your mental health

Any change can be hard to deal with. The death of my dad and my divorce were two of the hardest times of my life, and coming to terms with my deafness later in life was initially tough. It didn't help that these three life changes happened at once, like a queue of really shitty buses. Challenging moments can all come at once. I had to grieve the loss of my dad, my marriage and my hearing at the same time, which was very hard, but the grief process was a useful one. RNID advocacy officer Annie Harris advises: 'It's important to recognise that it is grief and it's okay to feel like the world has ended. But the end goal is acceptance: you just have to believe that it will happen one day, and be patient.' That's hard to imagine when you are curled up in your duvet in the dark, watering your pillow, but there will come a day when you will feel a little better. Amy Morton says:

> Take your time . . . be patient and kind to yourself. Allow yourself time to process the loss and allow yourself time to adjust to your hearing aids. Accept that it won't feel comfortable straight away, or it might do . . . Each person is so different in how they deal with change, so whatever is right for *you* is the right thing.

Amy is right that each person is different and your grief process might not start straight away; it might be years later. Many people don't view their deafness as 'a loss', but you might to start with. The loss that you feel in leaving your 'hearing' status behind will soon be filled with the joy, skills and experiences that being part of the deaf community will add to your life. Try to reframe deafness as a new addition rather than a subtraction. As Amy Morton says: 'Hearing loss for me now isn't a loss but something I have gained.'

If you are coming to terms with your new hearing aid or cochlear implant, Charlotte Hyde says: 'A bit of reassurance: no one cares. No one is looking at your hearing aid or cochlear implant. No one is judging you for being deaf. Even with twelve years of experience of communicating my deafness to others, I still stumble over this.' We are all more concerned with our own experiences – as we should be! So focus on you, and what you need during difficult times, rather than thinking about what the world might think of you. I know, it's easier said than done!

Mental health and your identity

'I know that I am different, that I am Deaf. I accept my identity, and I'm not going to change myself.' Thus, Deafhood was born and grew in a thousand little ways into a collective selfhood nurtured by a thousand little acts of rebellion, by a thousand and one little victories.

Paddy Ladd[79]

You don't need to change yourself for anyone else. Wearing a colourful hearing aid is an act of rebellion, speaking to a friend in BSL in a crowded cafe is an act of rebellion, and being happily deaf is an act of rebellion. And who doesn't love a rebel?! Rebel or stay quiet, you do you, but please never be ashamed of who you are.

Identity is very personal, and it's important to say that there is no one way to be deaf. 'Deafness isn't cut and dried or black and white. It doesn't exist in a binary. Deaf identity is fluid,' explains Charlotte Hyde. A lot of people struggle with this, as we don't have a lot of deaf role models in the mainstream media to take inspiration from. Audiologist Adam Chell says: 'It is difficult to generalise, but I find that the impact on self-image is a common theme.' If you have hearing loss later in life, it can challenge your view of yourself. You might think you know exactly who you are by your thirties, but a deaf diagnosis could change that. Who am I now? Am I disabled? How will this change my life? These are all questions I had when I discovered my hearing loss in my late twenties. I thought I'd done all my soul searching and trying on different versions of myself, but all of a sudden I was given new information that didn't necessarily fit.

245

A life change, like finding out you need a hearing aid or cochlear implant, doesn't just challenge your sense of identity, but having to wear the physical hearing aid or implant can highlight any existing issues you might have with your image.

Journalist Liam O'Dell explains:

> I was around thirteen or fourteen when I was told I might benefit from wearing hearing aids after undergoing a hearing test. Back then I was an incredibly self-conscious teenager with acne, whose self-esteem was pretty low, so the idea that I would have to wear two new things alongside my glasses, and run the risk of having people asking questions as to why I had two tubes poking out of my ears, terrified me. I grew my hair out so it could cover up my hearing aids. I think all of this was a mixture of anxiety over my own appearance, but also the fact someone might ask me a question about my deafness and my Deaf identity before I had found out the answers to these questions myself.

Those hormone-fuelled years are so important to our development and sense of self, and the way you view the world, so of course any extra challenges are going to feel overwhelming. I think it's important we acknowledge this to young people going through this process.

Founder of Deaf Identity Luke Christian says:

> Growing up, my deafness affected my mental health massively, because I found that everyone around me was always telling me how to act and behave as a deaf person – 'You can speak, so you're not deaf', 'You wear hearing aids, so

you are deaf'. 'How can you be deaf if you can't sign?' and 'I'm
fed up of repeating myself, turn your hearing aids up!' – so I
always struggled with my own deaf identity and which world I
belonged or fitted into, but now I realise it's not about trying to
fit in; it's about how I feel as a person with my own deaf
identity, and nobody can take that from me!

Discovering I was allowed to cultivate my own identity as well
as opinions on my own deafness and experience was a huge
turning point for me in terms of identity. I've been told by a
lot of people that I should call myself 'hard of hearing', but that
just doesn't resonate with me, and that's okay. There's no rush.
You can take your time to find out how you feel about your
deaf identity. Do what feels right for you.

For actor Sophie Stone her deafness has 'proven to be more
than an identity. It means visibility, strength, and existing
beyond low expectations and harmful tropes. It means
acceptance and finding joy.'

The stigma around premature ageing

When we're young, we all want to pretend we're older, closer
to adulthood, so we're taken seriously – and so we can get
into pubs and bars, if you were like me growing up. For me
the ages from eighteen to twenty-three meant free-spirited,
'living life' time, not worrying about my age or even thinking
much about it. From the age of twenty-four onwards, I started
worrying about getting old. I wonder if this happens earlier
for women because we are so judged on our appearances, but
I had a fear that time was running out. I remember noticing I
had eye wrinkles for the first time, getting my first grey hair,

the first time I stood up from a chair and groaned (it came surprisingly early for me), and I remember when I was told I had lost some hearing. Mark Atkinson says: 'We want to break down the stigma that hearing loss only affects older people, that there's nothing you can do about it and that you should keep quiet about it. Hearing loss can affect anyone at any time of their lives.'

Many people worry that wearing a hearing aid will be a visible signifier that they are ageing. I asked my mum about her hearing loss experience. Even though she was told she needed hearing aids in her mid-forties, she put off getting them until her early fifties. She said: 'I didn't want to be perceived as old before my time, and ever since I've had hearing aids, I wear my hair long to cover my ears.'

However, Amplifon audiologist Jane Noble says: 'I think untreated hearing loss will make you seem older than hearing aids will. People having to repeat themselves, the TV being loud, and responding inappropriately in a conversation seem more embarrassing to me.'

'If the wish to ignore deafness was not so pronounced, ear trumpets would be as common as spectacles,' said one farmer in Michigan in the USA in 1882 in Jaipreet Virdi's book *Hearing Happiness*.[80] Wow, right!? Almost 150 years later, we're still saying the same thing. Why do we want to hide any visible signs of deafness?

Jenni Ahtiainen, founder of Deafmetal, believes that: 'All beauty is in differences. Hearing aids are not just a clever innovation; they are also a way to show strength: this is who I am and I am lucky to have hearing aids.' In fact, when so many people across the world do not have access to hearing aids, we *are* lucky. We can also take pride in our deafness – and many young deaf people are leading the way when it comes to this. Whether this pride means wearing brightly coloured hearing aids or hearing-aid jewellery, opening up about their deafness or creating content on social media to raise awareness, the wave of Deaf Pride is growing stronger.

How to improve your mental health

While finding a community, having new experiences and a new passion have all had a positive impact on my mental health, one of the biggest positives for me is just knowing why I have struggled in hearing environments for so long.

Having an official diagnosis helped me by giving me permission to prioritise my experience and my mental health: to ask for support when I needed it, to say no to things. Also, finding out why you have been feeling socially anxious or isolated can be incredibly positive. If you have been blaming yourself for feeling uncomfortable in noisy party environments, discovering that you have hearing loss finally gives you something apart from yourself to blame, which can come as a huge relief. I always used to wonder why I avoided talking to people on the phone and why, as a teenager, my mum asking me to call the local takeaway with our order filled me with such dread. Looking back, I understand that I felt inadequate on those calls because I wasn't always able to understand everything being said, which made me feel bad about myself. Who knew failing at ordering a takeaway could be so important to a teenager?! Or maybe we did know, and that's why someone invented Deliveroo.

Audiologist Adam Chell explains: 'For some, being deaf is part of their identity. They don't see it as a loss. Think about how beautiful the world can be when you take away the din of traffic or crowded streets. They may notice the subtle details that hearing people miss. If an individual wears hearing aids, taking them off at the end of the day is the equivalent of throwing your shoes off your tired feet. Silence can also be their safe space for reflection and tranquillity.' In fact, Actor Sophie Stone loves 'the superpower to switch off and find complete zen, when no one who has hearing can'. Complete zen sounds like a pretty lovely mental state to me!

Illustrator Lucy Rogers reveals: 'I love how being deaf has helped make me into who I am now. I believe it has made me resilient, strong and open-minded. And of course, being deaf has led me to meeting my partner of eight years who is now my fiancé. He is deaf too, and I have many lovely deaf friends who I consider to be a second family.'

Finding a whole new support network of lovely people is definitely a positive, and can help you through the dark times.

It might take some time to get here, but many people I interviewed said they love being deaf. Loving something can have a huge positive influence on your mental health. Lucy Rogers advises us to 'make your deafness *your* strength. It makes you unique and different to others, which I think is so cool.' Actor David Bower explains: 'I think [good mental health] might be connected to having the right state of mind and having the right support structure around you, being secure in yourself and having self-belief, along with experience, education and knowledge.'

Your community

Something that can really help your mental health is support. There are lots of organisations that offer support online, via telephone and or text. Journalist Liam O'Dell says that the best thing about being deaf is 'Deaf culture. It comes with its own unique, visual language, and the talent of the deaf community is incredible.' Immersing myself in Deaf culture and the hearing loss community has really helped me feel supported and less alone. Liam advises:

> Find your community. There might be a Deaf club near you which you can join, or, if not, Deaf charities might be able to connect you with other Deaf people. There's also a strong deaf community on Twitter and Instagram. I'd encourage Deaf people to find whatever avenue is comfortable for them to express their Deaf identity, if that is what they want to do.

There is a strong black deaf community in the UK. The organisation Black Deaf UK provides resources and support via its Facebook group and social media accounts. Sarah Adedeji says, 'I love [the black deaf community]. It's probably the safest community I've been in.'

Reaching out to people on the same journey as you are is incredibly important. Sharing similar experiences, as well as learning from others in the community, is an invaluable tool – not just for your mental health, but also for your understanding of your own deaf experience.

Keighley Miles describes how it felt to connect with her local deaf community: 'Wow! These people understand what I feel and have had the same experiences as me, when I thought I was the only person who felt that way.' Annie Harris, RNID advocacy officer, explains that: 'I am part of Deaf culture, where I have a strong Deaf identity and accept being deaf. I have many wonderful deaf friends, and we attend many deaf-led events. I am lucky to experience this world, which I could not have if I were born hearing.'

Keighley Miles founded Families of Deaf Children to help deaf people feel less alone: 'I always make sure that the children all know that they are all equal and that the deaf community isn't just for the deaf person but also for the family of that person. They are involved just as much and, are just important.' She has succeeded in creating a supportive community – and the experience has also helped her personally:

> I had to fake being proud to be deaf to be a good role model for the children attending our events, but they turned out to be *my* role models. I can honestly say they make me smile and so proud every day, and their achievements mean as much to me as my own children's achievements. Seeing their faces when I take off my processor and say, 'Look, I'm the same as you', is priceless, and something that will never get old.

I was lucky enough to visit FDC in Essex to talk to the children and parents there (and sign a few copies of my children's books – ever the self-promoter), and I can attest to the incredible supportive, joyous atmosphere that Keighley and the other parents have created there.

Part 4
Support

Chapter 17
Am I disabled?

The word 'disabled' has an impact. Some people have very strong reactions to the word, whether good or bad. At first I struggled to think of myself as disabled, as a deaf person. I felt that others were *more* disabled than me, and I worried that if I called myself disabled it would somehow take attention away from other disabled people who needed support. I have come to realise that being disabled is not a competition! There are many types of disability, and all are valued. Legally, being deaf is recognised as a disability – and it was this legal status that helped convince me that calling myself disabled was 'allowed' and wouldn't disadvantage the wider disabled community. In fact, it was something as small as being eligible to apply for a Disabled Persons Railcard that helped me!

My experience is not the same as everyone else's, though. Blogger Bethan Harvey says: 'Yes, deafness is often referred to as a disability, but I don't see myself as disabled, nor do I see myself as any different from anyone else. My ears may not work but I can do anything and everything else anyone else can.' Actor David Bower, who uses BSL as his first language, says: 'In the deaf community, there was a felt experience of otherness from the disability scene owing to the language/ linguistic divide . . . yet I still feel a very strong connection to the disability community as a whole.'

Interior designer Micaela Sharp agrees: 'I would feel a fraud to say I was deaf or disabled because it implies you need assistance, and I don't often wear my hearing aid.' It seems there is a guilt that comes with having an invisible disability – as some would categorise deafness – as deaf people can 'pass' visually in an ableist world.

Another turning point for me was discovering that it wasn't me personally who was 'disabled' as a deaf person; it's society that disables people because it's not fully accessible. When I asked BSL user and actor Sophie Stone if she considered herself disabled, she said, 'Yes – disabled by society.' This is an important point, because then disability becomes more about accessibility and less about being singled out as people with something different about them. Journalist Liam O'Dell explains:

> While I agree with those who would argue it is just the case that our ears don't quite work and we are otherwise unaffected by society, we are indeed disabled by society when subtitles aren't available, venues don't book interpreters, and environments are loud and inaccessible to us. The view that it is societal attitudes and infrastructure which disables people is known as the social model of disability, and I apply this ideology to all of my disabled identities.

Research and speaking to the wider disabled community helped me have a better understanding of my disability, but for others it took a global pandemic. Amy Morton explains:

> Up until the pandemic, when people started to wear masks, I never considered myself disabled. I think this was as a result of the 'get on with it' approach my parents had – and there's

good and bad with that, I have to be honest. But when the pandemic hit and masks were introduced, for the first time I faced a constant barrier on a daily basis and it brought about unexpected anxiety . . . Out of what is challenging came huge growth, and so now I would say I have a disability. I now actively seek access and challenge getting my needs met. It's made me stronger to accept myself as a person with hearing loss. Yes, I have a disability – and it's a power!

Deaf historian and author Kathleen L. Brockway is passionate about this: 'We are always disabled. We are. We cannot say we are non-disabled. We need tools and resources to support our lifestyles. Unfortunately, I do not like the word "disabled"; I prefer to say I am deaf.'

Indeed, many people are proud of their deaf status and prefer to use this word, while still feeling they are part of the disabled community. However, Charlotte Hyde explains: 'You can be proud of being deaf while also identifying as disabled. There are plenty of disabled people who aren't deaf who identify as disabled and are proud to be so. Disability isn't a dirty word.'

Again, it is a personal choice. Being able to say 'I am disabled' has been a long journey for me. It's taken at least five years, I would say, but I now happily say that I have an invisible disability. However, often after you have made this choice you then have to defend it to others. There are still those who question my disability status – and the status of all deaf individuals. 'But you're not really disabled' has been a common response. It's tiring to have to stand up for yourself, and deafness as a whole, again and again to prove the ways in which society disables us from living. I was at a TV awards dinner recently, where I spoke to a TV director who said she was working on a new project with a channel that wanted to push disabled voices. I was excited that finally someone wanted to share our stories, and started to tell the director about my deaf journey. I had actually written a script where I, as a deaf person, and my friends, a charming deaf BSL speaker and a sassy wheelchair user, were enjoying living as single women in London, with all the adventures and sex that involves. The sex bit got her interest – it always does. TV people tend to love sex because it feels naughty – and who doesn't like a bit of naughty, right?! However, she told me that I would have to write the script from the point of view of the wheelchair user because I – as a deaf person – wouldn't fit the brief. I took a deep breath and asked her to clarify what she meant. She looked me up and down, laughed uncomfortably and said, 'Well, you're not disabled, are you?'

No one can tell you how to identify, particularly not a non-disabled person. I am sorry if the same thing has happened to you too, because it's not nice.

The language to use

If you use identity-first language, this means you say 'disabled person'. If you use person-first language, you'd say 'person with a disability'. But which should you use?

Identity-first language is generally preferred by the disabled community, so it should be your default when referring to disabled people. Often the abled argument is 'I see the person, not the disability.' This isn't the compliment some people think it is. If someone has to use person-first language to emphasise that a disabled person is a person, there's something very wrong that goes deeper than language. Disability is often a huge part of our lives and it's not shameful, however much society tries to stigmatise us.[81]

The Purple Pound

So you have decided that you're disabled, but what next? You could support disability charities, communities and voices as well as disabled people in your workplace. And here are some facts you can tell businesses to encourage them (they shouldn't need encouragement, but they usually do) to become accessible for staff and customers alike.

In the UK, it is thought that some 7 million people of working age [are disabled], which adds up to an awful lot of spending power. This is known as the 'purple pound' and [in 2017] was reckoned to be worth around £249 billion to the economy.[82] More than 1 in 5 potential UK consumers has a disability.[83]

- Businesses lose approximately £2 billion a month by ignoring the needs of disabled people.

- The spending power of disabled people and their households continues to increase. In 2020 it was estimated to be worth £274 billion per year to UK businesses.

- 73 per cent of potential disabled customers experience barriers on more than a quarter of websites they visited.

This advice is taken from the Inklusion Guide, an incredible resource for the publishing industry written and researched by Julie Farrell and Ever Dundas.

You can find more information and excellent advice relating to accessibility at www.inklusion.org.

Chapter 18

What *not* to say to someone with hearing loss

All the things in this chapter have been said – repeatedly – to me and to the other deaf people I interviewed for this book. 'What not to say to someone who is deaf?' is the most common question deaf people get asked, and the pressure to constantly educate hearing people is immense. So this chapter is for all deaf people, so we don't have to answer this question any more: everyone can just read the below and get the lowdown. The key point? As actor Sophie Stone puts it: try 'not being a dick, helps massively.'

'You don't look deaf' or 'You're too pretty to be deaf'

Founder of Living with Hearing Loss Amy Morton says, 'Please never say "you don't look deaf" – what is that supposed to mean?!' Blogger Bethan Harvey thinks it's strange too:

> I'm not quite sure what a deaf person is supposed to look like. Am I supposed to be green and slimy, have ten heads, no ears (well, I'm halfway there with that one), have 'I'm deaf' tattooed on my head? I've no idea, and of all the deaf friends I have and deaf people I've met, I can honestly say there isn't a look. We're human – we look like average, typical people because that's exactly what we are.

If you're talking about being too pretty to be deaf – well, some of the hottest people are deaf (and yes, I include myself among them). Other hot deaf people include Halle Berry, Marlee Matlin and all the people I interviewed for this book.

'It doesn't matter'

This is one of the most common phrases that deaf people and people with hearing loss get, and it's also one of the most frustrating. Amy Morton explains, 'Please don't ever say "I'll tell you later" or "Never mind, it wasn't important." That's so hurtful, excluding and just belittling . . . I want to understand you!'

If someone can't hear what you've said and you reply with 'It doesn't matter', you are excluding the deaf person. It does matter. Inclusion matters. Yes, even if you were saying something silly or telling a rubbish joke, let us understand it first and then we can decide whether it matters or not. If all it takes to include someone is repeating your sentence, then isn't it worth it?! Would it really put you out that much?!

'I'm so sorry'

If someone decides to trust you by telling you they are deaf, do not reply with the above. We don't want pity. Usually we're telling you so you know how to communicate with us, or we're telling you that we're deaf as it's one of the things that make us who we are (like my love of knitting, my obsession with Nando's sauce, and my comedy skills).

Author Kathleen L. Brockway declares: 'I wish they would stop feeling sorry for us. They always say "OH, I'M SO SORRY" when I say I'm deaf.'

'I wish I could learn sign language'

Then do. If you were saying 'I wish I could go to the moon', I'd want you to believe in yourself, but that might be a little harder to achieve. It's relatively easy to learn BSL, so don't wish – just do! As Kathleen L. Brockway says: 'I don't want to hear it. I want them to do it and learn, then they can come up and talk to me in sign language.'

'You can speak, so you're not deaf'

First of all, no one can tell you how you should identify your deafness. They can let you know that a lot of people call themselves hard of hearing, for example, but that doesn't mean *you* have to call yourself hard of hearing. Moreover, a hearing person shouldn't offer you their opinion on whether you're deaf or not, unless they are your audiologist, and even then they don't always get the terminology right.

When it comes to speaking, blogger Bethan Harvey explains:

> Some deaf people choose to speak, while others choose not to. A lot of it is down to personal preferences about how the individual wishes to communicate. It can depend on the level of access to speech and sounds too. The most important thing is we all have a voice; we just use it in our own ways. It doesn't make anyone's voice any more or less important than anyone else's.

'You don't sound deaf, you speak so well'

When someone 'sounds deaf', this is called the 'deaf accent'. Not all deaf people have this. Bethan Harvey explains: 'It depends on the level of sound access a deaf person has. I am forever being told I drop my vowels (a, e, i, o and u) when I'm talking, especially when I'm tired. This is purely because I can't hear these sounds in words. It's harder when I'm tired – listening fatigue and trying harder to concentrate, to ensure I'm speaking correctly, take its toll.'

If, like me, you discovered your deafness later in life, your oral language will have developed before your deafness. People often say I 'speak well for a deaf person', but lots of deaf people speak without a 'deaf accent' – and who is to say that speaking 'well' means speaking without an accent? Also, having a deaf accent does not indicate your level of deafness. For example, some people with profound deafness will have no accent, whereas some people with moderate hearing loss will have an accent.

'You are deaf, do you read Braille?'

Bethan Harvey explains:

> Believe it or not, Braille is not used by the deaf – unless of course they are deafblind. One of the librarians at our local library got excited a few weeks ago. She came up to me and said, 'Oh, was it you who ordered the Braille books? You're the only person I know that signs.' I wasn't rude, but I quickly corrected her that Braille is, in fact, for the blind, not the deaf, and that deaf people can read,

'Deaf people suffer from their condition' or 'Samantha suffers from hearing loss'

Blogger Bethan Harvey says: 'Deaf people do not suffer; it's not a debilitating illness, it's not a life sentence. Deafness is just a different ability and a different way of life.'

Deafness is not a disease. It is not being deaf that makes us suffer; it is the barriers society puts in our way that cause suffering.

'How can you be deaf if you can't sign?'

In the UK roughly 150,000 people communicate using BSL compared to the 12 million people in the UK who are deaf or who have some form of hearing loss. So, in fact, the majority of deaf people don't sign.

'You're wearing hearing aids, so you're deaf'

As we explored, the terminology around deafness and hearing loss can be extremely personal – and political. Many people who wear hearing aids are happy to call themselves deaf, like me, while others feel uncomfortable with the label of deaf, and many deaf people don't wear hearing aids at all. So hearing aids do not always equal 'deaf'. It's important to be led by the individual.

'I'm a bit deaf'

Bethan Harvey argues:

> No, you're not a 'bit deaf', you've just misheard or missed something. Don't try and play the deaf card to make us feel

265

better. It doesn't. This is totally different from actually being deaf. I don't know if it's supposed to be a way of being reassuring or trying to be understanding and helpful, but it's really not. Sorry, but you're either deaf, have hearing loss, or you don't. We don't wake up and decide 'I might be a bit hearing today.'

If you would like to relate or connect to the deaf community, listen to us; don't try to pretend that you're one of us.

'You can't be deaf – only old people are deaf'

Well, this is just factually incorrect. Some old – or 'older', as my mum prefers me to say – people are deaf due to noise-induced hearing loss over time. However, many children are born deaf and I discovered my deafness in my late twenties. As Bethan Harvey explains: 'Deafness can – and does – affect anyone of any age at any time in life. Yes, it can be true that hearing deteriorates with age, but it doesn't mean that is the case for everyone.'

'Are you actually properly deaf, though?'

This is a strange one. I think what people are trying to ask here is if I am profoundly deaf. The level of someone's deafness can be very personal – it's not something that you need to ask. How deaf we are isn't a competition, and doesn't take anything away from other deaf people's experiences. If our level of deafness affects our accessibility needs, we will tell you, or you could ask if there is anything you can do to help, but asking any more than that is an invasion of our privacy.

'You are not disabled'

If someone identifies as disabled, then they are. It's not up to you to tell them whether they are allowed to identify that way or not. Deafness is legally recognised as a disability, so deaf people are 'allowed' to call themselves that from a legal standpoint. However, many people would rather call themselves deaf.

'My grandad is deaf'

Great, but it's unlikely that I know him, if that is what you're suggesting. This is a bit like me telling you I'm bisexual and you telling me that you know someone else bisexual. We don't have a big bisexual WhatsApp group (although I kinda wish we did).

Bethan Harvey says: 'My reaction would be "That's nice . . . I'm not quite sure how I'm supposed to feel or respond to you telling me your grandad is deaf." Is this suggesting that deafness is an older-generation problem?'

'Hearing aids cure deafness'

This is incorrect. Hearing aids amplify sound. Bethan Harvey explains: 'Hearing aids, as the name suggests, are aids. They do not cure deafness, and nor do bone-anchored hearing aids, cochlear implants, or bone conduction implants. With or without them, you are still deaf. There is no cure.'

267

'Deaf people are "stupid"'

Not true. Intelligence and deafness are not linked. While inaccessible education settings may hinder a deaf person's access to education, we are not 'stupid'. I mean, have you read all the words I put together in this book? This association of being deaf and 'stupid' is a historical hang-up from generations of mistreatment of deaf humans, when deaf people were ignored, not deemed worthy of education, sent to asylums or even killed. This stereotype is steeped in misunderstanding, prejudice and cruelty. After all, Beethoven was deaf and he was a musical genius. Just imagine – if he'd been ignored or hidden from the public consciousness, we would have lost so much.

'Hearing loss and deafness only affects your hearing'

As this book has explored, hearing loss and deafness can impact your life in a number of ways, including your emotions, your mental health, and at work. There are so many positives to being deaf and having hearing loss. Unfortunately there are negatives too, mainly due to accessibility issues put in place by the hearing community.

What you should say

Me: 'I am deaf and wear a hearing aid.'

You: 'Oh, cool. I follow brilliant deaf content creators on Instagram. Hermon and Heroda, their handle is @being__her – do you follow them?'

Or

You: 'Thanks, I appreciate you letting me know. Do tell me if there's anything I'm doing that could be more accessible for you. [Facing me with mouth clear and speaking normally] Do you want a drink?'

Or

You: 'I wasn't aware of that – thank you for telling me.'

Or

You: 'Wow. I know some deaf people use BSL – do you? I am currently learning myself from an awesome Deaf instructor.'

Or

You: 'Yes, I know. I've read your book and it's really opened my eyes. I shall now leave it an excellent review online.'

Chapter 19

How can you support deaf people?

This chapter is all about how hearing people can be allies to people who are deaf or have hearing loss.

'I'm a business owner – how can I help?'

You can employ deaf people and create accessible work environments for Deaf and disabled people. See Chapter 12 for more information on working with hearing loss and deafness.

'I am a cafe/restaurant/bar owner – how can I help?'

Founder of SoundPrint app Gregory Scott advises: 'For restaurants, lower the background music, get acoustical treatment, add plants, drapes, tablecloths for better sound absorption/reflection. Educate the public and venue managers on the dangers of excessive noise exposure.' Also employ deaf people – this one is a recurring point!

'I am a performer/theatre company/theatre venue – how can I help?'

Employ deaf people.

Don't just think about what might work *for* deaf people; work with us creatively as well as on accessibility. Just think about all the creative ways we have had to come up with to navigate a hearing world: wouldn't you love to work with our creativity?! Angela Barnes also advises: 'If you really want to make your shows accessible to the deaf community, you could both caption a show and have a BSL interpreter.'

'I am a teacher – how can I help?'

If there are any deaf children at your school, then you should be provided with deaf awareness training (I think all teachers should have this anyway). Learning some basic BSL from a registered provider like Signature is a great start. You are the gateway to an amazing education for so many deaf children, and educating hearing children about deafness, hearing aids and hearing loss can make your class a much more welcoming environment for deaf pupils. Deaf awareness classes, learning BSL together, inviting deaf speakers into the class, reading books with deaf protagonists, learning Deaf history, learning how hearing aids work when you learn how the ear works – all these can contribute to a full education for deaf and hearing students alike.

Making sure your lessons are accessible is very important. Having written instructions is useful so there is no confusion: face the class when speaking so children can lip-read (no turning to the board to write while talking); provide deaf students with class materials ahead of time/afterwards to review in case they missed anything in class. Adjusting the seating arrangements in class can also make a big difference to lip-reading: sit deaf children closer to the front (without singling them out) and space out the tables so they can lip-read other children. Create an acoustically pleasant environment with sound-absorbing materials on the walls/ceiling and soft furnishings to help reduce background noise. As you are a teacher, you can have fun with this and work with the children to create an environment they are proud of and can help to make with you. Get some large sheets of fabric or old curtains and ask the children to add drawings to them (perhaps of themselves and their classmates) using fabric pens, then hang the curtains on the wall. Children could learn to sew (yes, both sexes) then they could pick out a cool fabric and make their own cushions for a reading area. Use old clothes/fabric to create sound-insulating panels as a class, to encourage recycling. We know how hard teachers work already, so thank you – I hope these ideas help to spark your own ones!

'I run a school – how can I help?'

Welcoming deaf children and providing an accessible environment is so important, as is educating your hearing children. Organising deaf awareness training for all staff members is a great start. NDCS provides a free CPD-accredited 'Introduction to Deaf Awareness' course via its online training portal,[84] which would be a brilliant start. There are lots of free resources on the NDCS website, and NDCS also provides £20 training workshops online. You should be able to contact your local authority for funding around accessibility too. Providing BSL lessons for staff, parents and students would be brilliant, as would looking at the layout and acoustic set-up of all communal areas, as above (this includes staffrooms, as you may have deaf members of staff too).

NDCS says: 'Since 1 September 2014 the Children and Families Act 2014 has had a big impact on the way children and young people aged 0–25 with special educational needs and disabilities (SEND) are supported in education. This means that: Local authorities (LAs) must set out a "Local Offer" of the support they expect to be available for children and young people with SEND in their area. Schools and nurseries must publish a SEN information report on their website and update it each year. These reports should explain how the school or nursery has put their SEND policy into practice.'[85]

Employ deaf people! If you have deaf pupils, letting them see deaf role models in their learning environment can be life-changing. Consult with parents and children at your school about their individual needs, and champion the voices of deaf and disabled people.

'I am a deaf person – how can I help?'

It is important to say that you can be deaf and get on with your life. Please don't feel obligated to educate others and be a spokesperson for the community if that doesn't feel right for you. However, if you feel that you want to take a stand then sharing your experience is always welcome. RNID chief exec Mark Atkinson says: 'Having successful, funny, loud voices showing the way forward is really important.' So why not volunteer with a charity, get involved with your local community, fundraise for a local Deaf school, or become a leader in your field of work and act as a role model for other deaf individuals? You could also become a leader in *a* field, but I think that's called being a farmer, which is also valid.

'I am a hearing person – how can I help?'

'I think hearing people just need to think more about deaf awareness. It's very low down as an issue in our national consciousness, which is astonishing when you consider the number of people directly or indirectly affected,' says Mark Atkinson. 12 million people in the UK have some form of hearing loss or deafness – yes, I'm repeating that statistic again, but it's an important one! Chances are, you know one of those 12 million, but maybe they haven't opened up to you yet for whatever reason. Avoid speaking *for* deaf people but be a hearing ally: read literature by deaf people (hi!), support deaf business owners, take part in deaf-focused projects for the greater good, educate yourself on deafness and hearing loss and its impact and, I will say it again, EMPLOY DEAF PEOPLE.

'I'm an architect – how can I help?'

You can actually help and make a huge impact on deaf people's lives without sacrificing a building's structural integrity or beauty! Making buildings accessible starts at the design stage. When drawing up your design, ensure that doors are wide enough for wheelchairs, don't have steps up to all the entrances, have accessible toilets and lifts, and think about sound-absorbing building materials and room shapes. If you are creating a room with high ceilings, add a design feature that will help absorb the sound so the room isn't echoey. If you are designing offices, create breakout spaces that can be a respite from open-plan areas. Insulate your walls properly so that sound doesn't travel from room to room. Think about noise pollution from your building, after it is made and while it is being built. Use sound-absorbing materials wherever possible.

Also . . . employ deaf people.

'I'm an interior designer – how can I help?'

You can put soft furnishings everywhere. I imagine those are the words you've always wanted to hear? Curtains, cushions and upholstery all absorb sound – and look stylish while doing so. Let's have all the layers and patterns, plants, creatively sectioned-off areas and soft fabrics, please.

'I'm an audiologist – how can I help?'

Listen to your patients – ironic, I know. Know the science, yes, but know the social and mental impact of deafness too, and have support materials available. Listen to the deaf community about terminology/tech advancements/culture as well as listening to the big hearing-aid corporations. Remember, we are human beings too.

'I'm a GP – how can I help?'

Create an accessible practice and be deaf-aware. Allow patients to book appointments via text/email. Have screens to notify patients in the waiting room. Remove masks while talking. Keep your mouth clear and face the deaf person. You might not be in charge of all of these things, but making everyone in your practice aware of them will make a difference. Keep yourself up to date on language around deafness, and champion deaf colleagues.

'I'm a writer – how can I help?'

Write about deaf characters and include deaf experiences. Work with deaf writers to inform your work and support the work of deaf writers.

'I'm a work colleague – how can I help?'

Be deaf aware and encourage your employers to get deaf awareness training for the whole staff. Be an ally for your colleague – ensure their accessibility requests are heard and implemented. Think about accessible meeting spaces, presentations, etc. Make sure any video content is subtitled and any audio content is transcribed. Listen to your deaf colleagues and follow their lead (e.g. don't out them as deaf to every new person you meet).

Don't take it upon yourself to educate your workplace; this should be done by a qualified professional.

'I'm a friend – how can I help?'

Take some responsibility for finding accessible environments where you can meet deaf friends. Research quiet restaurants/venues to invite your deaf friend to, ask venue managers to turn down background music, create an acoustically pleasant environment in your own home. Be deaf aware, know how to be a good lip-speaker, and learn BSL.

'I'm a human being – how can I help?'

You can support deaf-led projects/campaigns/business and actually LISTEN (yep, it feels ironic to write that) when deaf people tell you about their experiences and how you can do better.

You could also support a deaf-focused charity. Charities like RNID are striving to make society more accessible for deaf people. Mark Atkinson listed the charity's achievements, from

277

'successfully lobbying the NHS for free hearing aids back in 1948, through to hearing screening for newborn babies in 2000. In 2022 we we've been part of an amazing coalition of charities that successfully fought for BSL to be made an official language of England, Wales and Scotland.'

You can find more charities and organisations to support in the resources section.

Chapter 20
In the media

As one of the few British deaf presenter/actor/comedian/broadcasters/authors, I'm lucky enough to be asked to do some amazing things when deafness comes up in the media. I – along with a select group of D/deaf activists – seem to be the go-to person to be called to comment on deaf issues. I'm not complaining – we all need a job. My work as an actor means that I'm also called on when deafness is portrayed in a film or a TV programme, and I've been honoured to interview some of the key creators of deaf content in the media over the last few years. I believe that asking a deaf person to interview other deaf people is excellent: it brings a new insight to an interview that might otherwise be very stereotypical if it was conducted by a hearing person with little knowledge of the deaf community. I would encourage all media outlets to have more disabled presenters and inter-viewers on their talent lists. We can, of course, present and interview on other subjects that aren't determined by our deaf-ness or disability. What I'm basically saying is: give us more work, please.

Before working in the media, my knowledge of deaf represent-ation in TV, film and literature was very narrow – non-existent, even. There has always been *some* deaf and disabled representation, if you search for it, but very little in mainstream media. If a deaf influence is there, it is often ignored. Nyle

DiMarco talks about deaf influences on one of the first famous film stars, Charlie Chaplin, in his book *Deaf Utopia*:

> Off-screen, Chaplin enjoyed collecting art, and one of his favourite painters was a Deaf man named Granville Redmond. The two men became friends, and Chaplin valued Redmond's art so much he set up a studio for Redmond at his lot in Los Angeles. Later, Redmond would go on to appear in a few of Chaplin's movies . . . In some movies, Chaplin even went so far as to actually use ASL signs.

It feels huge to find out about this deaf influence on Charlie Chaplin, who so many people cite as one of the first comedians. When I look back at my own comedy, I can see why I quite often leaned towards the visual, performing 'act outs' rather than just using my words. I remember my first experience of performing stand-up comedy on the radio: it was a large tent at the Edinburgh Fringe Festival with a live audience, and the audio was being recorded for Radio 4. In the run-up to the gig I remember trying to craft some of my best material into a tight seven-minute slot and realising that so much of it, since it was visual, wouldn't work on the radio. I had a bit about Sally Ride – the first American woman to be sent to space. She was up there for seven days. The story goes that the engineers at NASA asked her if one hundred tampons would be enough . . . for seven days! That's not even the joke; that's just the true bit. I then had some act-outs about what she'd do with all the tampons, including shooting them out of her vagina like a tampon machine-gun while shouting 'Next!' If you imagine me thrusting my vulva at an audience over and over with sound effects, you might understand just how visual my comedy can be.

TV and Film

Deaf and disabled voices and influences have been ignored for decades, and it's exciting to see so many new perspectives being spotlighted. I hope in the future we see even more deaf and disabled viewpoints and representation in the media. And these people don't have to be there purely to talk about disabled issues. I'm excited to see deaf/disabled representation where the people included are living full, happy lives, not always being oppressed and facing some kind of injustice. (Although, to be fair, we do have to deal with a lot of that.) Stories that raise awareness of accessibility, oppression and that educate are incredibly important, but so are stories of joy (which avoid pandering to a non-disabled or hearing audience).

My first memory of seeing a deaf person in the media was in the film *Four Weddings and a Funeral*, directed by Richard Curtis. Deaf actor David Bower played Hugh Grant's deaf brother, David. Even though he had a small role in the film, it was an impactful one. It was the first time I had seen sign language actually in a drama, instead of via an interpreter in the corner of the screen. I was delighted that David's character was treated 'normally' by everyone else in the film, and I wanted to see more of his life. David Bower is still an actor, and he runs Signdance Collective, an interdisciplinary performance collective. He told me: 'When I realised that you didn't have to be a hearing person to be an artist, that excited me, and I immediately started exploring ways to get involved.'

David was very kind when I met him, and smiled all through my stilted BSL (it can take years to become fluent, and I'm still learning) and apologies. He signed:

I was very young when [*Four Weddings*] was made, and it was quite hard to understand how to follow that through and get more film work. I tried to muddle as gracefully as I could through the ensuing commotion surrounding the publicity machine and hype and the pressure that brings. Almost thirty years have passed since and it has receded to a quiet memory. We recently made a short for Comic Relief and it was nice to catch up with everybody again.

Are things any better now? Why is deaf representation so important?

Role models

I'm passionate about the importance of representation in the media for people who are deaf, people with hearing loss, Deaf culture, deafblind people, LGBTQIA+ deaf people and deaf people of colour.

Victoria Sylvester, who teaches at a specialist school for deaf children, says that: 'Students in our school often feel "different" and try to hide their deafness, especially as they become teenagers. Being represented means that they can look up to people who are admired and respected, and in turn feel respected in mainstream society themselves.'

One of the UK's most famous deaf actors is Sophie Stone:

I've built a name and paved paths for others, so even if it all stops now, I can say I left the door open. I didn't pull up the ladder. I trusted there'll be more spaces at the table, and I was part of that change. My deafness has given me an edge:

the fire I needed to keep trying, a unique journey into the
world of acting, writing, directing, consultancy work, teaching,
translating, creating and existing as exactly who I am – while
also being a million characters to dive into. In this job, there
will never be a day where you don't have to prove yourself,
but at least now it's getting easier to do that without also
having to prove that 'Deaf Can'.

Sophie has done such amazing work, but this important issue
can't all be on the shoulders of one talented woman. We need
the people in charge to push representation too – that means
TV commissioners, publishers and heads of companies. As
Clare-Louise English says of current representation, there is
'not enough variety and nuance. People are not just Deaf or
hearing, there is sooo much in between – that's where I exist
and what I love to explore in my work.' Claire-Louise is co-
founder and co-artistic director at Hot Coals Productions,
which creates theatre and independent film work. There does
seem to be better representation in these areas. There have
been recent shows at the National Theatre, the Soho Theatre
and touring shows that seem to explore the breadth of deafness,
but this is something we need to see reflected in mainstream
media too. Rose Ayling-Ellis gave the Alternative McTaggart
lecture at the Edinburgh TV Festival in 2022, which was
covered widely in the UK press. In it she said: 'I am done with
being the token deaf character. I believe that diverse, rich and
fascinating deaf stories are ready to go mainstream and that we
can do this together.'[86] To this I say YES! I totally agree – but
will anyone listen?

Keighley Miles from FDC believes it is already happening. She
says: 'I'm so excited for the next generation of deaf adults,

because I know these children are going to build on the success of people like Rose from *Strictly Come Dancing* and change the world for deaf people and show the world we are proud and not shy to shout about our achievements.' Luke Christian, the creator and owner of clothing brand Deaf Identity (as worn by Rose Ayling-Ellis on *Strictly*) is one of the people doing great things in the media to combat stereotypes. He says: 'When I grew up, deaf people were always portrayed in a "woe is me" way, or we were shown that deafness only affects people through old age, which isn't the case at all. So I wanted to create a strong fashion brand that felt modern, fresh and fun by breaking down old stigmas and barriers surrounding the deaf community.' Things are happening – but is it enough? Illustrator Lucy Rogers thinks: 'People are now talking more about deafness. It's lovely to see and I still think we need a *lot* more. There are so many talented deaf people, and it would be great to showcase them as well.'

Actor Nadia Nadarajah believes things are getting better: 'Now, in 2023, it has gotten better – but have we "cured" it and reached peak representation? No. There is still a long way to go.' She goes on to explain her positive experience working on TV show *Vampire Academy*: 'They saw me like a normal person and oh, we just need to bring in an interpreter. So that's been great. I was pleased to have an opportunity to meet the writer. The writer knows about language, and we're working in to another language, considering how that works parallel to the filming process.' This joined-up thinking, working with the writing team and having an interpreter on set is what I would like to see more of!

In August 2022 Mattel released a Barbie doll with a hearing

aid – or, as I affectionately call her, deaf Barbie. This isn't the first doll to have a hearing aid or cochlear implant, but it's the first to be mass marketed. It was promoted by Rose Ayling-Ellis, who said, 'We're getting rid of that narrative of what is beautiful.'

Leading Deaf news blog Limping Chicken reported:

> The actor now hopes toy brands will represent a 'different range of Deaf people', including different races, cochlear implant users, Deaf people with multiple disabilities and BSL signers. Calls for more toys representative of disabled people have been made in the past through the Toy Like Me campaign – founded by deaf writer and journalist Rebecca Atkinson. The project has already created Deaf dolls, with a Deaf Tinker Bell wearing a pink cochlear implant going viral in 2015.[87]

It is amazing to have this representation for children, who can play with a doll that looks like them, and I hope this is the start of lots more toys of this type. I also hope this means the company is addressing accessibility for their staff and customer services, rather than this just being a front-facing push.

Advocates can be role models outside the mainstream media too. Instagram and TikTok especially are becoming incredible platforms for talented deaf people to spread their messages to a wider audience. Just check out these people: @signkidgram, @justmecameil, @being__her, @mrlukechristian and @liamodelluk.

Policy change can also provide political role models. The 'Subtitle It!' campaign I am involved with, backed by RNID, has received press recognition and thousands of signatures in an online petition shared on social media. Changing the law with the BSL bill has seen a real change for Deaf BSL users, as Annie Harris, RNID advocacy officer, explains:

> The process of the BSL bill becoming an Act has created much public awareness, in part thanks to Rose from *Strictly Come Dancing* and increased representation on TV and films. This is wonderful, and I am already seeing more people signing 'thank you' or practising deaf awareness around me. I am genuinely excited at what the future could bring.

CODA

CODA stands for child of deaf adults, and it's also the title of a film that made waves (good and bad) – in the deaf community and the hearing community – around deafness. Starring Oscar-winning Marlee Matlin and Troy Kotsur, the film depicts a Deaf family with one hearing child, played by Emilia Jones. An independent film, first shown at the Sundance Film Awards, *CODA* was picked up by cinemas worldwide and won countless film and media awards, culminating in making history by winning Best Picture at the Oscars. This film came at a time when deafness had finally been brought on to the global agenda by other films and activists, but it's arguably *CODA* that has put deaf actors and representation on the map.

I was lucky enough to be asked to interview the cast of *CODA* for Apple TV and RNID. Sometimes it's useful being a deaf girl in the media industry, as I get cool opportunities like these. For our interview with the deaf cast of the film, we had BSL interpreters for the British audience and ASL interpreters for the cast, as they were American. It felt joyous to be a deaf person interviewing other deaf people, and being given the platform to do that. While I'm not a CODA, I could relate to some of the struggles depicted in the film – and as an actor, I was thrilled to hear about the accessibility on set. One of my favourite moments in CODA is when the hearing daughter is singing to Troy Kotsur's character and he puts his hands against her throat to feel the vibrations. There is also a moment in the film when the deaf family members turn up at the school gates listening to loud music in the car, and Troy's character says something about enjoying the vibrations of the music against his balls! I think what this film managed to do was bring humour to stereotypes of the deaf experience, which illuminated the truth within them. Troy Kotsur was truly deserving of his Oscar and other award wins: director Sian Heder really allowed his acting talent to shine. It's beautiful to see a deaf actor being given the space to not only act but also use sign language to add to character nuance and humour. Troy's performance is a masterclass in comedy acting for both hearing and deaf audiences alike. I would recommend watching this film for Troy's performance alone, but it also happens to be very good, so you'll enjoy it for its content too. It is worth pointing out that the film received criticism from some in the deaf community for its audist lines, music and deafness obsession, and the idea that CODAs are 'suffering' by being born into a deaf family. As Liam O'Dell writes for the Limping Chicken, '[the CODA character] appears to be held back by her own Deaf family – and yes, that's as problematic as it sounds.'[88] While it is important to remember this is a representation of one fictional family's story, there is a problem when it is the only representation that most people will see. The portrayals in the film could misinform many people about what it is like living with a deaf family, if they take it to be 'the norm'. I think the important thing is to have more representation and more films like this, to represent a range of stories.

Sound of Metal

As a deaf girl in the media world I was also delighted to be asked to interview the director of the movie *Sound of Metal* for the British Film Institute. The hearing director, Darius Marder, explained his connections to the deaf community which informed the film as well as explaining his choice of using a hearing actor for the main role. Riz Ahmed plays a character who loses his hearing quite suddenly and is launched into the deaf community in an environment where his peers only sign in ASL. There is a depiction of cochlear implants and incredible achievements in sound to depict his deaf experience. I feel it's the closest a film has got to audibly conveying how being deaf might feel. There was some backlash from the deaf community due to the director's choice of using a hearing actor, and the negative portrayal of cochlear implants, though.

Children's books and representation

When I was growing up I loved to read. I loved immersing myself in the world of books, and my mum says I was often so wrapped up in a book that I didn't hear her calling me for dinner. Now we know I might not have heard her calling for dinner for another reason, but I still absolutely love to read. However, in all the books I read throughout school and sixth form, I never read a book with a deaf character. I don't mean a deaf main character, I mean any representation of a deaf character: no deaf friends, sidekicks, chance acquaintances with deaf people . . . No deaf representation at all. When I was young I also loved to write short stories: one of my stories was even chosen and put on the board at my primary school, which was a proud moment. However, I never believed I would be an author. I came from a middle-class family who came from a working-class background and I was the first person to go to university in my family – then I studied drama, so what a disappointment that was! Seriously, though, my family were very supportive of my dreams of being an actor (also, drama is not the easy degree you might think it is), and even though I enjoyed English and Classical Civilisations at A Level, I never believed I could be good enough at writing to be paid to do it for a living one day. So the idea of writing a book seemed like a distant dream that only really clever people or really posh people could achieve. (It's funny when people say I'm posh now because I never see myself that way. That's what drama training does to you, dahling).

How I wrote my first book

When I found out I was deaf and I got my hearing aid, I started to work with RNID as a volunteer ambassador and began to engage with other deaf individuals and families. Often I would be asked if I could recommend any media or books with good deaf representation that families could watch or read together. At the time I realised that, even though I was now an adult, I had still never read a book with a deaf character. Maybe I've just been reading the wrong books, but there it was. So I began to search for deaf representation in books. I found *El Deafo*, an excellent graphic novel for children by Cece Bell with a deaf main character. Hurrah! It's a great book and I still recommend it, but for years it seemed like the only book out there.

As I began my deaf journey I searched for more books that could help me sift through all the information out there about hearing aids and deafness and what it was like to live as a deaf person in modern society. I found scientific textbooks and academic essays, which were incredibly interesting but which took time to understand and wade through. I took to social media to find my peers who might be able to explain what living with deafness and hearing loss was like in a more accessible, fun way. Listen, I know that scientists and academics are also fun, so there's no judgement or criticism here, but I wanted to hear personal stories of hearing-aid fittings, mis-understandings caused by deafness, and feeling frustrated by the ableism in society and not knowing what to do about it.

I decided that maybe I could write a book, and it would be for people like me, who wanted to know what it was like to live with hearing loss and deafness but who didn't want to wade through lots of academic texts to get there. I thought it could be funny and honest, and it would have some proper facts in it too, but no one wanted me to write that book. I didn't know how the book world worked at that point, so I wrote up a pitch document like you do for telly and I sent it to a few publishers that I'd met on Twitter. Most didn't reply, but those who did said there was something in it and they liked my writing, but then the correspondence seemed to dry up. There didn't seem to be any enthusiasm for this type of book, so I let that dissuade me.

I was still really keen to improve representation for people with hearing loss and deafness, and that's when I met a children's publisher called Knights Of, whose remit was diversity in publishing. The first time I met Dee Stevens, one of the founders of Knights Of, I told them I didn't want to write children's books. Dee wasn't put off talking to me after my declaration, and let me know a bit about publishing and writing in the children's books world. Dee had a sense of humour, which helped. After that meeting I couldn't get the idea of children's books out of my head. I suddenly thought that maybe there would be a market for a children's book with a deaf main character. Maybe it was in this industry that I could try to help with representation – and have fun doing it (I do love a fart joke, and luckily children like them too). I messaged Dee on Twitter and asked them if they'd be interested in working on the children's book with me. Dee asked what it was about, and I explained the importance of deaf represent-ation, together with things I was interested in, like space and space travel, and came up with an idea. Dee told me to go off and write it because it sounded interesting, and in my naiveté I took that as a book commission. No contracts or money had changed hands, but I was convinced that my book was going to happen.

That was how my book *Harriet Versus the Galaxy* began. It was published by Knights Of and it is a book about Harriet, a little girl with a hearing aid that translates alien languages, and she and her gran protect the Earth from aliens. The book is an adventure story at its heart, with fart jokes, as I promised, aliens with two bottoms, aliens who eat socks, and even knickers – and most importantly, deaf representation. Harriet tells readers about her hearing aid, how she got it, how she maintains it, and the sounds she hears – all while fighting off aliens. It was a pretty fun book to write, and I still can't believe

Knights Of published it with the tiny amount I knew at the time about children's books. But they did. That book opened my eyes to what representation can do in people's lives.

I've had letters from parents of deaf children and deaf children themselves thanking me and explaining how funny and important they found the book. Children with hearing aids have brought the book into school so that their class can understand what living with hearing aids is like. Teachers have purchased a book for their school to help children with hearing aids and deafness feel seen among their classmates, and to start conversations about deaf awareness in school. I've been sent pictures of little girls with hearing aids dressing up as Harriet in *Harriet Versus the Galaxy* for World Book Day, and showing off their hearing aids with pride. I also now go into schools whenever I can to talk to children about the book and hearing aids and deafness and what that means, as well as telling even more fart jokes, and I can honestly say it's one of my favourite things to do. To date, writing *Harriet Versus the Galaxy* is one of my proudest moments because of the massive response the book has had within the deaf community. I'm proud to be able to offer some representation, even if it is informed by my own individual experience. I've since written another book, called *The Night the Moon Went Out* (published by Bloomsbury Education) about a little girl called Aneira. She wears two hearing aids that she takes off to charge at night, and she's scared of the dark because the dark can be extra-scary when you can't see and you can't hear.

I was honoured when this book was longlisted for the inaugural Adrien Prize 2023, a prize for commercial children's fiction that explores the disability experience.

I would encourage any deaf writers who would like to write a novel with deaf representation to go for it. While it can be useful at times to be one of the few deaf authors writing deaf characters, it would be lovely to have some author friends and to be able to represent more deaf experiences informed by deaf authors. The more the merrier!

So how did I end up writing *this* book? Well, after the success of my children's books I came back to this idea of writing a funny, honest guide to hearing loss and deafness, the book I wanted to read when I got my hearing aid. Again, I was told that this book was niche and people didn't know if it would sell, but due to the increased representation and success of so many deaf people in the industry, like Rose on *Strictly* and Nyle DiMarco in America, there was interest from one publisher. So thank you to Headline for not dismissing this book as niche. Thank you from the 12 million people in the UK who have some form of hearing loss or deafness. Whether or not they read the book, they might feel for a moment that deaf people have at least a tiny glimmer of representation in literature. It's so exciting to see the new wave of deaf and disabled voices sharing their stories through fiction, non-fiction, television and film. Let's do more of it. Let's focus on a new generation of deaf voices – and that doesn't just mean young voices, it means *new* voices, whatever their age or experience. If you are reading this and have always wanted to write a book, play, TV show or film, but because you're deaf you feel like people won't want to see it, let me tell you you're wrong. We want you, we want you to do the thing you love, and we want to hear your story. It's important. It's needed. I can't wait to see it.

While there are more children's and young adult books with deaf characters now, there are still only a few written by deaf authors. Here are some of the other children's books with deaf representation by deaf authors:

Can Bears Ski? by Raymond Antrobus (Walker Books, 2022)

Major and Mynah by Karen Owen (Firefly Press, 2022)

Set Me Free by Ann Clare LeZotte (Scholastic, 2021)

Show Me a Sign by Ann Clare LeZotte (Scholastic, 2020)

The Silence Between Us by Alison Gervais (Blink, 2019)

True Biz by Sara Novic (Little, Brown, 2022)

The Reckless Kind by Carly Heath (Soho Teen, 2020)

FAQs

These are questions that I, and other deaf people, get asked a lot. I also put out a call on my social media for people to suggest any questions they'd like answers to, and so a lot of those are included here too.

Is hearing loss reversible?

No. Once you have an official diagnosis of hearing loss, then your hearing will not return or 'get better'. The only time your hearing could get better is if you have a blockage like ear wax, which can be removed.

So I have hearing loss. Where should I start trying to understand this new experience?

Well, after getting advice on whether a hearing aid/cochlear implant would work for you, the RNID website (https://rnid. org.uk/) has lots of tools and resources that will help. Hopefully this book will help too. Seek out other deaf people in your area, by looking up local deaf groups on the internet (Facebook is particularly good for this) or signing up to a local BSL class where you could meet other people at the beginning of their journey.

What does BSL stand for?

British Sign Language.

Do deaf people use Braille?

No, Braille is a type of raised writing that you read by feeling. It is used by people who are blind.

What does CODA stand for?

Child Of Deaf Adult.

Can deaf people drive?

This is the most googled question when it comes to deafness and hearing loss! Yes, deaf people can drive. It is totally legal and there are no extra tests or equipment that you need to drive when deaf.

Are there cost implications with hearing loss/deafness for adults?

Yes. While you can get a hearing aid and batteries on the NHS, many people (who can afford it) choose to go private. A single hearing aid can cost up to £3,500. Hearing assistance devices such as flashing alarms, doorbell systems, BSL interpreters, speech-to-text apps, transcriber apps, learning BSL, etc., also cost money. Only one cochlear implant is funded on the NHS for adults, so if you choose to have a second implant, that can cost you thousands. There is some help available: you can apply for disability benefits, but this will depend on your personal situation. You can also apply for a Disabled Persons

Railcard, which gives you one-third off rail travel. But unfortunately, yes, it is expensive to be deaf.

What does ASL stand for?

American Sign Language.

Does your inner ear feel different when you go deaf?

No. Unless you go deaf because of something that causes pain, like a burst eardrum or an infection, there is no inner ear 'feeling' that will tell you that you have gone deaf. I think this is partly why it takes people so long to do anything about signs of hearing loss, because there is no physical feeling to act as a marker.

Can people with hearing loss enjoy music?

Yes, absolutely. Lots of deaf people can still hear music – we might miss certain lyrics or music at high or low frequencies, but we can still enjoy music. Profoundly deaf people might not be able to hear much of the music, but can still enjoy music environments like gigs for the atmosphere, and they can enjoy music through vibrations.

Can deaf people read?

Er, yes. I'm deaf and I wrote a book for other deaf people, so… However, if BSL is your first language then you will be used to a different sentence structure than written English. That's why, when communicating in written form with BSL users, it is best to stick to precise, clear sentences and avoid idioms.

Can deaf people have sex?

Oh yes, and we do.

What does SSE stand for?

Sign-Supported English.

Will hearing aids interfere with my ear piercings?

It depends on the type of hearing aid you get. Behind-the-ear hearing aids won't touch or interfere with lobe piercings, whereas cartilage ear piercings could knock a behind-the-ear hearing aid (depending on the size of your ear in relation to the hearing aid). An in-ear hearing aid would not come into contact with lobe or cartilage piercings, although it could touch a tragus or daith piercing, as could a behind-the-ear hearing aid, due to the tube that goes into your ear. It also depends on the type of hearing aid and ear mould you have. Blogger Bethan Harvey explains:

> I have multiple piercings in my left ear, three in my lobe, one in my helix and one in my daith . . . it doesn't seem to be an issue. My hearing-aid tube just avoids touching it. The tubing on my hearing aid is very thin and flexible . . . My hearing aid slightly touches the back of my helix piercing where it hooks over my ear, but doesn't seem to be an issue and doesn't give me any discomfort or feedback issues.

Is deafness contagious?

No, not at all. It can be hereditary, but you can't catch it. It's not a cold or a ball.

What is Deaf Havana?

An English rock band from Norfolk. Yes, seriously.

Are deaf people attractive?

Yes! Check out my picture! Being deaf doesn't affect your appearance – other than the possible addition of a hearing aid.

Are you worried about passing on the deaf gene to your children?

No, because I don't view deafness as a negative. I understand the ways I can help make the world more accessible for them, like BSL and the deaf community, and so I am happy for any child I might have to be hearing or deaf.

What other books can I read?

I recommend books written by D/deaf people, such as *Deaf Utopia* by Nyle DiMarco, *I'll Scream Later* by Marlee Matlin and *Hearing Happiness: Deafness Cures in History* by Jaipreet Virdi in non-fiction. Also *True Biz* by Sara Novic, *El Deafo* by Cece Bell, *Can Bears Ski?* by Raymond Antrobus and my children's books, of course: *Harriet Versus the Galaxy* and *The Night the Moon Went Out*. I was also proud to write a piece for deaf poetry anthology *What Meets the Eye?* (published by Arachne Press). For poetry, try *Deaf Republic* by Ilya Kaminsky, and the poetry of Meg Day is sublime.

So do people who use BSL as a first language not use hearing aids?

Yes and no. There is no rule to this; it is down to the individual.

Yes, some people who are told by an audiologist that they would benefit from using a hearing aid choose not to have one. But some do: actor David Bower, a BSL user, says, 'I wear hearing aids and have done since I was diagnosed as Deaf when I was a child.'

Where can I keep up to date on deaf news stories?

LimpingChicken.com: the UK's independently run deaf blog and news site

Hearinglikeme.com: a news and lifestyle website for people whose lives are affected by hearing loss

Liamodell.com: an award-winning freelance journalist and campaigner specialising in deafness, disability and social media

I am waiting for my hearing aids to be fitted. What can I do in the meantime?

RNID advises:

> If you are waiting for your hearing aids to be fitted, you could try other equipment to help you hear better. Assistive listening devices[89] are portable amplifiers that you can use to hear sounds more clearly. They are good for listening over background noise or from a distance. You could also try learning some communication tactics[90] with the people in your household. These include learning to lip-read, asking people to get your attention before they start talking to you and asking people to speak slower if you need them to.[91]

It's really important that you wait for your fitting and don't try to buy any hearing aids second-hand and fit them yourself, as you really won't get the proper benefits from them.

How do I change my hearing-aid batteries?

You should be shown how to do this at your hearing-aid fitting, but, as I mentioned earlier, mine was a total blur and I didn't retain much information from it! You can ask your audiologist to show you at your next check-up, but YouTube is a great resource – would you believe it? If you search 'How to change your hearing-aid battery' there are lots of useful videos that will guide you through the process, step by step. You don't need to find a video showing your specific hearing aid, as the process is pretty much the same for all sizes of battery. It can be fiddly, but stick with it – soon you will be a pro!

> **Top tip**: turn your hearing aid off before changing the battery to avoid it whistling in your hands.

How do I change the tubing on my hearing aid?

So, listen, I didn't know this was a thing, but apparently the tubing needs changing every four to six months. Although if there are no blockages and your hearing aid is still working, it should be fine. I just leave mine until my next audiology check-up and then ask for advice.

If you do need to change your tubing, RNID has a handy leaflet available via its website, Adjusting-to-your-hearing-aids-leaflet. pdf (see p. 314), that contains a step-by-step guide. Or you could search 'how to change a hearing-aid tube' on YouTube for some really useful videos. Some hearing-aid providers also offer a postal repair service. Or you could speak to your GP, as the NHS provides local hearing-aid clinics too.

I am hearing muffled sound through my hearing aids – what should I do?

If you can, contact your audiologist to book an appointment, or contact your hearing-aid provider, who may be able to talk you through any steps to correct the issue, or may offer a postal repair service.

The RNID website suggests some common reasons you may be hearing muffled sound:

If you're having trouble hearing things with your hearing aid, you should check:

- that the hearing aid is fitted comfortably
- that the hearing aid is switched on properly
- the volume control on your hearing aid, if it has one
- that you haven't switched your hearing aid to the hearing loop setting by accident
- that there isn't moisture or wax in the tubing
- that the ear mould or soft tip (if your hearing aid has one) isn't blocked with ear wax
- to see if the wax filter needs changing, if you have an in-the-ear or a receiver-in-the-ear hearing aid
- that the battery is the right way round, or needs replacing[92]

Are there any deaf brands I can support?

Yes! Here are some.

Deaf Identity is a deaf-owned clothing brand created by Luke Christian: www.deafidentity.com

Creative greetings cards: https://elizabethmugridge.co.uk/

Little Auricles is a hearing-aid jewellery company set up by an audiologist based in Australia: www.littleauricles. com/au

Maddy Studio on Etsy for beautiful sign language greetings cards: https://www.etsy.com/uk/shop/maddystudiouk

Hitcreations4U on Etsy (set up by the mother of a Deaf child) for personalised BSL products

Deafmetal is a deaf-owned hearing-aid jewellery brand based in Finland. It was founded by Jenni Ahtiainen: https:// www.deafmetal.store/

Worldwide Deaf Gym: https://worldwidedeafgym.com/

Iceland tours, Iceland: https://m.facebook.com/deaficeland tours/?ref=page_internal

Online interior design and decorating services in America: https://www.jjonesdesignco.com/

Girl & Creativity, America (ASL): https://www.girland creativity.com/

Benefits support and LGBT+ inclusion training: www. wheeliequeer.net

Lucy Rogers is a deaf illustrator and has illustrated books including *What Does a Beaver Do?*, *What Does a Bee Do?*, *Adventures with Hank and Louie: The Christmas Witch*, *The Quest for the Cockle Implant* and *The Night the Moon Went Out*.

Penguin in the Room is an award-winning arts marketing company owned by a deaf individual (yup, that's me again): https://www.penguinintheroom.com/

Food, drink and restaurants

Yumma Food, a catering company set up by Yvonne Cobb that also runs cooking classes taught in BSL: http://www.yummafood.co.uk/

Maharajah Coffee, London and Kenya: https://maharajahcoffee.com/

The first deaf-owned restaurant in Belgium, Soepbar Sordo, Ghent: https://visit.gent.be/en/eat-drink/soepbar-sordo

Bravo Cafe, Taipei, Taiwan: https://www.tripadvisor.co.uk/Restaurant_Review-g293913-d12940201-Reviews-Bravo_Cafe_Taipei_Nangang_Shop-Taipei.html

The first deaf-owned restaurant in Paris, 1000&1 Signes, France: https://www.1000et1signes.com/

Tapas restaurant L'Oreille Cassee, Toulouse, France: https://loreillecassee-toulouse.com/

An American brewery set up by three Deaf guys, graduates of Gallaudet University: https://www.streetcar82brewing.com/

Restaurant chain Crepe Crazy, Austin, Texas, USA: https://
www.crepecrazy.com/#about

ASL pasta: https://shop.parentsgonehiatus.com/en-gb

You can also support deaf writers, film-makers and content creators by watching, reading or interacting with – and, importantly, sharing their work.

You can also support the Samantha Baines brand by buying my children's books and merchandise.

Acknowledgements

Well, what a journey writing this book has been! Thank you to everyone who has ordered it, bought it from a bookshop, read it and shouted about it – it honestly means so much. Books by deaf and disabled authors don't always get as much press as other books, or don't even get commissioned in the first place, so please don't stop here: keep sharing, recommending and supporting other deaf and disabled authors.

There have been so many utterly wondrous people who have helped this book come to fruition. First, my brilliant literary agent, Jo Bell at Bell Lomax Moreton, who has been so kind, supportive and funny, and who totally believed in my potential to write a book, even when I didn't! Hannah Layton, my glorious manager, thank you for sticking with me for so many years and through so many different career branches. Thanks to the marvellous Lindsey Evans at Headline, my editor, who gave me confidence in my writing for possibly the first time ever (yes, I realise I have published two other books already, but hello imposter syndrome!). Lindsey, thank you for having faith in my idea, and me, and thank you for being so committed. To the fabulous team at Headline: Kate Miles, Isabelle Wilson and Jane Hammett, who guided me through copyedits, cover design, page proofs and press – thank you. Kate, you'll never know how much your email saying 'the lawyer found your book completely fascinating' cheered me up.

To the wonderful people I interviewed for this book – thank you, and thank you again. Thank you for sharing your experiences so openly and replying to all my emails, especially the ones saying 'I just wondered if you'd had a chance to look at my email yet . . .' A special thank you goes to all the BSL signers, who even translated their answers into written English for me – you went above and beyond! A massive hello to the 'deafie crew' – you know who you are, and our WhatsApp group is the most supportive, informative place.

A special mention must go to Charlotte Hyde. I'm sorry I interrogated you over coffee in Hyde Park, but thank you for helping me to work through my ideas and giving me the lowdown on deaf academia. Liam O'Dell, I am honoured that you agreed to be my sensitivity reader, and I am so appreciative of all the work you have done as a journalist and a champion for deaf people. Thank you.

Adam Chell, my audiologist – thank you for looking after my ears and letting me send you random hearing-aid questions via Instagram. To all the excellent charities mentioned in this book that have created a wealth of online resources, thank you – and please continue your incredible work. RNID, thank you for having me as your ambassador for so many years, and for welcoming me and including me in your campaigns – it has brought so much joy and positivity to my deaf experience. Particular thanks go to Lucy Devine at RNID, who always answers my emails, even the one I sent at 1am asking her to confirm a statistic!

Mum, to whom this book is dedicated, who has hearing aids like me, and just got on with it for so long without kicking up a fuss until I got my hearing aid and created a big old fuss – I love you. I'm sorry you had to 'carry on' for so long with minimal support, and I am so lucky to have you in my life. Thank you to my sister, Emily, who is creative and passionate and constantly keeps me grounded by telling me 'you are not famous' if I'm ever called 'a celebrity' in the press. Thank you to my partner for taking the dog for walks after a long day at work so I could finish my edits.

Finally, thank you to my old GP for sending me for a hearing test 'just in case'. You started this whole journey, and I'm not sure I would have gone for a hearing test if it hadn't been for you. Thank you for noticing the signs, even when I didn't, and for taking the time to refer me. You'll never know how much you changed my life that day.

List of resources

Here's a list of websites that provide support:

RNID: www.rnid.org.uk

Deaf Unity: https://deafunity.org/

Signature: https://www.signature.org.uk/

Black Deaf UK: www.facebook.com/BlackDeafUK/

Tinnitus UK: https://www.tinnitus.org.uk/

British Deaf Association: https://bda.org.uk/

National Children's Deaf Association: https://www.ndcs.org.uk/

Deaf Rainbow: https://deafrainbowuk.org.uk/deaf-lgbt-history-uk/

Helpful books, articles and links

Books

Nyle DiMarco with Robert Siebert, *Deaf Utopia: A Memoir – and a Love Letter to a Way of Life* (William Morrow, 2022).

Sarah Novic, *True Biz* (Little, Brown, 2022).

Jaipreet Virdi, *Hearing Happiness: Deafness Cures in History* (The University of Chicago Press, 2020).

Paddy Ladd, *Understanding Deaf Culture: In Search of Deafhood* (Multilingual Matters, 2003).

Articles

Howard Alexander, 26 November 1998, 'Hearing aids: smaller and smarter'. The *New York Times*: https://www.nytimes.com/1998/11/26/technology/hearing-aids-smaller-and-smarter.html

Boots Hearingcare, 'How do hearing aids work?': https://www.bootshearingcare.com/hearing-aids/how-do-they-work/

Gil Kaufman, 'Will.i.am reveals he has tinnitus, ringing in the ears'. MTV.com, 7 December 2021: https://www.mtv.com/news/wdh90c/william-reveals-he-has-tinnitus-ringing-in-the-ears

Amazon Hearing, 'Communicate and stay connected with Alexa': https://www.amazon.co.uk/b/?node=21730997031

Apple, 'Accessibility: Hearing – catch every word, sign, or signal': https://www.apple.com/accessibility/hearing/

Deaf Unity, 'About us': https://deafunity.org/about-us/

Deaf Unity, 'How is deafness affecting your mental health?' https://deafunity.org/article_interview/deafness-and-mental-health/#:~:text=In%20the%20deaf%20community%2C%20worryingly%20this%20number%20rises,to%20experience%20mental%20health%20issues%20than%20hearing%20people

BBC News (2019), 'Cochlear implants to benefit more people with hearing loss': https://www.bbc.co.uk/news/health-47475036

Naomi Clarke, The *Independent*, 'Rose Ayling-Ellis urges TV channels to 'fix problem' and subtitle all shows': https://www.msn.com/en-gb/lifestyle/style/rose-ayling-ellis-urges-tv-channels-to-e2-80-98fix-problem-e2-80-99-and-subtitle-all-shows/ar-AA117LmU

Links

Connevans: a source of equipment and audio products for deaf people: https://www.connevans.co.uk

Otter.ai (voice meeting notes and real-time transcription): https://otter.ai/

Disabled Persons Railcard: disabledpersons-railcard.co.uk

Louder than Words – workplace assessments: https://louderthanwords.org.uk/workplace-assessments/

NHS website: acoustic neuroma: https://www.nhs.uk/conditions/acoustic-neuroma/

Makaton: https://makaton.org/TMC/TMC/About_Makaton/Who_uses_Makaton.aspx

DeafSpace | Gallaudet University: https://gallaudet.edu/campus-design-facilities/campus-design-and-planning/deafspace/

Handspeak, 'Deaf people driving on the road': https://www.handspeak.com/learn/index.php?id=280

Useful articles by RNID

Information and support: https://rnid.org.uk/information-and-support/

Types and causes of hearing loss and deafness: https://rnid.org.uk/information-and-support/hearing-loss/types-of-hearing-loss-and-deafness/

Cochlear implants: https://rnid.org.uk/information-and-support/hearing-loss/hearing-implants/cochlear-implants/

Making conversations clearer: https://rnid.org.uk/information-and-support/technology-and-products/making-conversations-clearer/

What to do if you're waiting for hearing aids to be fitted: https://rnid.org.uk/information-and-support/hearing-loss/hearing-aids/what-to-do-if-youre-waiting-for-hearing-aids-to-be-fitted/

Adjusting to your hearing aids: https://rnid.org.uk/wp-content/uploads/2020/04/Adjusting-to-your-hearing-aids-leaflet.pdf

What to do if your hearing aids need adjusting or repairing: https://rnid.org.uk/information-and-support/hearing-loss/hearing-aids/what-to-do-if-your-hearing-aids-need-adjusting-or-repairing/

Endnotes

1. https://www.thebsa.org.uk/public-engagement/faqs/
2. Nyle DiMarco, *Deaf Utopia*, p. ix.
3. https://www.who.int/teams/noncommunicable-diseases/ sensory-functions-disability-and-rehabilitation/highlighting- priorities-for-ear-and-hearing-care
4. https://rnid.org.uk/information-and-support/hearing-loss/ types-of-hearing-loss-and-deafness/genetic-hearing-loss-and- deafness/
5. https://www.who.int/news-room/fact-sheets/detail/ deafness-and-hearing-loss
6. Jaipreet Virdi, *Hearing Happiness: Deafness Cures in History*, p. 1.
7. S.G. Curhan, A.H. Eliassen, R.D. Eavey et al., 'Menopause and postmenopausal hormone therapy and risk of hearing loss', *Menopause*, 2017 24(9): 1049–1056. doi: 10.1097/ GME.0000000000000878.
8. https://rnid.org.uk/information-and-support/hearing-loss/ types-of-hearing-loss-and-deafness/ototoxic-drugs-and- hearing-loss/
9. https://rarediseases.org/rare-diseases/acoustic- neuroma/#:~:text=An%20acoustic%20neuroma%2C%20 also%20known,hearing%20and%20balance%20(equilibrium)
10. https://www.nhs.uk/conditions/hearing-loss/

315

11. https://www.nhs.uk/conditions/glue-ear/
12. Jaipreet Virdi, *Hearing Happiness: Deafness Cures in History*, p. 33.
13. https://www.nhs.uk/conditions/hearing-aids-and-implants/
14. https://www.bootshearingcare.com/hearing-aids/how-do-they-work/
15. https://www.apple.com/uk/accessibility/hearing/
16. https://rnid.org.uk/information-and-support/hearing-loss/hearing-implants/cochlear-implants/
17. https://www.bbc.co.uk/news/health-47475036
18. https://www.nhs.uk/conditions/hearing-aids-and-implants/
19. Jaipreet Virdi, *Hearing Happiness: Deafness Cures in History*, p. 23.
20. Ibid, p. 76.
21. https://www.nytimes.com/1998/11/26/technology/hearing-aids-smaller-and-smarter.html
22. Ibid.
23. https://www.express.co.uk/life-style/health/1648067/samantha-baines-hearing-loss-deafness-tinnitus
24. Jaipreet Virdi, *Hearing Happiness: Deafness Cures in History*, p. 4.
25. https://makaton.org/TMC/TMC/About_Makaton/Who_uses_Makaton.aspx
26. https://deafunity.org/article_interview/international-sign-language/
27. https://atlalipreading.org.uk/your-questions-answered-2/
28. https://atlalipreading.org.uk/your-questions-answered/
29. https://lipspeaker.co.uk/
30. https://www.stagetext.org/for-venues/theatre-captioning/
31. https://www.stagetext.org/for-venues/theatre-captioning/
32. https://www.stagetext.org/for-venues/theatre-captioning/
33. https://rnid.org.uk/information-and-support/technology-and-products/making-conversations-clearer/
34. https://www.amazon.co.uk/b?ie=UTF8&node=21731044031

35. https://www.amazon.co.uk/l/21731042031
36. https://www.amazon.co.uk/l/21731052031
37. https://999bsl.co.uk/about/
38. https://otter.ai/
39. https://www.connevans.co.uk/catalogue/106/Phonak-Roger-Radio-Aids---Hearing-Aid-Accessories
40. https://www.ndcs.org.uk/our-services/services-for-families/apply-for-a-grant/
41. https://www.tinnitus.org.uk/pages/faqs/category/what-is-tinnitus
42. https://www.mtv.com/news/wdh90c/william-reveals-he-has-tinnitus-ringing-in-the-ears
43. https://www.tinnitus.org.uk/pages/faqs/category/what-is-tinnitus
44. https://www.theguardian.com/lifeandstyle/2018/feb/12/seven-ways-to-deal-with-tinnitus
45. https://learningjournals.co.uk/benefits-of-sign-language-in-child-development/
46. https://www.nhs.uk/conditions/hyperacusis/
47. https://www.nhs.uk/conditions/hyperacusis/
48. Jaipreet Virdi, *Hearing Happiness: Deafness Cures in History*, p. 3.
49. Sara Novic, *True Biz*, p. 30.
50. Ibid, p. 32.
51. https://www.ncbi.nlm.nih.gov/pmc/articles/PMC5292361/#:~:text=Far%20peripheral%20vision%20plays%20a,but%20not%20central%20visual%20stimuli
52. https://gallaudet.edu/campus-design-facilities/campus-design-and-planning/deafspace/
53. https://www.soundprint.co/venue-managers-tips
54. https://wfdeaf.org/our-work/human-rights-of-the-deaf/
55. https://www.msn.com/en-gb/lifestyle/style/rose-ayling-ellis-urges-tv-channels-to-e2-80-98fix-problem-e2-80-99-and-subtitle-all-shows/ar-AA117LmU

56. https://rnid.org.uk/information-and-support/communication-support/

57. https://rnid.org.uk/information-and-support/technology-and-products/

58. https://rnid.org.uk/information-and-support/your-rights/your-rights-at-work/

59. https://deafunity.org/article_interview/deafness-and-mental-health/

60. https://www.ndcs.org.uk/about-us/news-and-media/latest-news/deaf-pupils-achieve-entire-grade-less-at-gcse/

61. https://limpingchicken.com/2022/03/29/single-send-system-proposed-by-uk-government-as-it-finally-publishes-education-review/

62. https://didlaw.com/disability-discrimination-solicitors-london/disabilities/deaf-discrimination-at-work

63. https://www.lawsociety.org.uk/topics/client-care/providing-services-to-deaf-and-hard-of-hearing-people

64. www.inklusionguide.org

65. https://louderthanwords.org.uk/workplace-assessments/

66. https://louderthanwords.org.uk/workplace-assessments/access-to-work/

67. https://www.gov.uk/access-to-work

68. https://www.gov.uk/access-to-work

69. www.inklusionguide.org

70. Jaipreet Virdi, *Hearing Happiness: Deafness Cures in History*, p. 2.

71. https://www.bbc.co.uk/news/blogs-ouch-29846154

72. https://rnid.org.uk/information-and-support/benefits/armed-forces-compensation-scheme/

73. https://www.cityam.com/tube-drivers-get-ear-defenders-for-screeching-underground-lines/#:~:text=Transport%20for%20London%20(TfL)%20has,their%20union%20threatened%20a%20strike

74. https://www.disabledpersons-railcard.co.uk/

75. https://www.handspeak.com/learn/index.php?id=280
76. https://www.tinnitus.org.uk/
77. https://www.bbc.co.uk/news/disability-35762887
78. https://deafrainbowuk.org.uk/
79. Paddy Ladd, *Understanding Deaf Culture: In Search of Deafhood*, pp. 314–15.
80. Jaipreet Virdi, *Hearing Happiness: Deafness Cures in History*, p. 73.
81. www.inklusionguide.org
82. https://www.bbc.co.uk/news/av/business-39040760
83. https://wearepurple.org.uk/the-purple-pound-infographic/
84. https://www.ndcs.org.uk/our-services/services-for-professionals/training-courses/e-learning/introduction-to-deaf-awareness-cpd-accredited/
85. https://www.ndcs.org.uk/information-and-support/education-and-learning/getting-additional-support/getting-additional-support-england/support-for-special-educational-needs-and-disabilities-send-in-your-area/
86. https://www.msn.com/en-gb/lifestyle/style/rose-ayling-ellis-urges-tv-channels-to-e2-80-98fix-problem-e2-80-99-and-subtitle-all-shows/ar-AA117LmU
87. https://limpingchicken.com/2022/08/16/rose-ayling-ellis-on-new-deaf-barbie-doll-were-getting-rid-of-that-narrative-of-what-is-beautiful-anymore/
88. https://limpingchicken.com/2021/08/18/liam-odell-coda-blames-deaf-people-for-societys-inaccessibility-and-its-damaging/
89. https://rnid.org.uk/information-and-support/technology-and-products/
90. https://rnid.org.uk/information-and-support/hearing-loss/living-with-hearing-loss/communication-tips/
91. https://rnid.org.uk/information-and-support/hearing-loss/hearing-aids/what-to-do-if-youre-waiting-for-hearing-aids-to-be-fitted/

92. https://rnid.org.uk/information-and-support/hearing-loss/hearing-aids/what-to-do-if-your-hearing-aids-need-adjusting-or-repairing/

Index

Index